TRACTION

The Neuroscience of Leadership and Performance

Accelerate your leadership with NeuroTREAD™

Kristen Hansen

First published by Kristen Hansen – October 2017

Kristen Hansen
Mobile: +61 414 504 797
Email: kristen@enhansenperformance.com.au

Author: Hansen, Kristen
Title: TRACTION – The Neuroscience of Leadership and Performance
ISBN 978-0-957-8089-4-2

Edited by Michelle Phillips

Cover design by Jesus Cordero

Text design by Rod Mercier

Typeset by Mercier Typesetters Pty Ltd, Telopea NSW

Printed in Australia by Griffin Press, 168 Cross Keys Rd, Salisbury South SA

ABOUT THE AUTHOR

Kristen Hansen

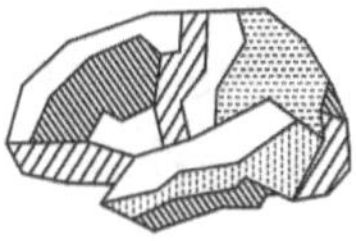

Kristen Hansen is the founder and CEO of EnHansen Performance, providing leadership development solutions via training, speaking and executive coaching. Established in 2003 following twenty years as a sales manager for various large Australian organisations, Kristen has specialised in programmes developing managers in the neuroscience of leadership and performance.

Kristen has always been interested in human potential and leadership. She is fascinated by the latest brain research on how to excel in these areas.

She is also accredited in PRISM Brain Mapping, the world's first online neuroscience based assessment tool, and is a master trainer and accredited practitioner in Emotional Intelligence with Genos International.

With a Post Graduate Certificate in the Neuroscience of Leadership from Middlesex University in the UK, a Bachelor of Business from UTS, Sydney, and a Diploma in Human Resource Management from Monash University, Victoria, in addition to her senior sales leadership experience, Kristen has a wealth of experience and knowledge on business, people and how the brain works.

Kristen developed the NeuroTREAD™ framework model to apply the findings from the field of neuroscience into relevant leadership and development topics. NeuroTREAD stands for how to Think, Regulate, Engage, Adapt and Develop with the brain in mind. Her main mission is to improve leadership capability at all levels of management. By understanding the mechanics of the brain, managers can engineer their own change and support change in others.

Kristen is a coach, trainer and speaker, servicing organisations in finance, telecommunications, technology, manufacturing, services and government. She has trained and presented her NeuroTREAD model to over 7,000 managers, and licenses the programme to organisations and consultants. Kristen has delivered her programmes throughout Australia, New Zealand, Asia and the United States.

NAVIGATING TRACTION

The Neuroscience of Leadership and Performance

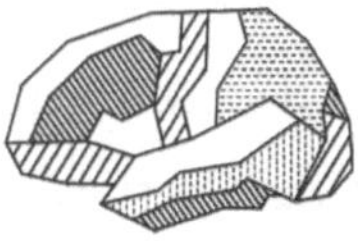

For context, the first chapter of this book outlines the challenges that are faced by managers and those in human resources and learning and development roles in organisations today.

The following chapters cover the NeuroTREAD framework – how to THINK, REGULATE, ENGAGE, ADAPT and DEVELOP with the brain in mind. Each chapter contains some sub chapters.

The largest chapter is the first one, THINK. We examine some of the key relevant brain structures in this section, before looking at some of the aspects of decision-making and insights.

REGULATE covers three key areas: How to regulate emotions and a 30-second circuit breaker, how to renew our cognitive and creative abilities, and how to build resilience on a daily basis.

The first two areas of THINK and REGULATE focus on a manager's ability to lead themselves well. This includes learning how to maximise cognitive and creative abilities to achieve good outcomes, decisions, and creative directions, as well as being able to remain calm under pressure, bounce back after set-backs and enjoy a healthy work-life balance.

ENGAGE then moves on with how to improve engagement levels. Understanding that engagement is a measure of emotional contribution measured in the effort and commitment a person has to a role, we look at a few of the things that managers can do to build engagement with their team members. First we look at the role that emotion contagion makes, and then look at the social motivators that shape a person's emotional responses to another in a social context. We also look at high performance from an individual and team perspective and what we can do to move up the performance curve.

ADAPT looks to understand how the brain changes. It discusses how we can use neuroplasticity – the brain's ability to change and form new habits – to improve the performance of ourselves and others in our team. By understanding how the brain has some natural resistance to change, but also understanding how the brain can be rewired, everyday high performance habits can be formed.

We next look at how managers can lead through change and the concept of 'Adaptive Leadership'. This is a need for leaders to be agile and adaptive, to create an environment and conditioning for others where change is an accepted norm and a place where people thrive.

DEVELOP is the final chapter of the book. This chapter looks at how we can develop others through a brain-based coaching approach. Utilising the neuroscience of goal setting, insights, the sub-conscious and likelihood of commitment to actions, the chapter explores the GROW-WISE model of coaching. This takes the well-known GROW model of coaching and puts a brain-specific lens on the best way to help people get from where they are now to their desired outcome. This can be utilised in five minute conversations where someone may be stuck on how to move forward regarding a challenge, through to an ongoing coaching and performance series that develops team members over a period of time.

In the last few pages we'll cover the key insights I've made over the last 10 years working with executives through coaching, training and leadership keynote presentations, and my thoughts on where the focus will continue from here.

Contents

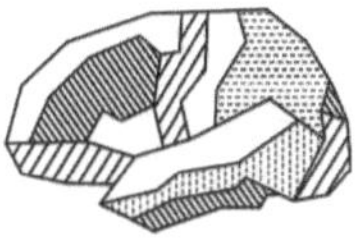

PART TWO
REGULATE

PART THREE
ENGAGE

PART FOUR
ADAPT

INTRODUCTION

The Challenges Facing Leaders Today

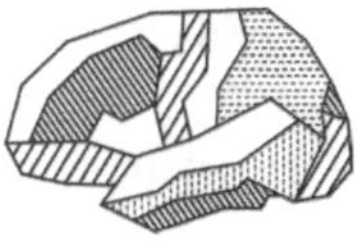

Neuroscience is transforming leadership development. When I refer to leadership, it is important to think of both self-leadership and leading others. Without effective self-leadership, we can't be effective leaders of others.

Our core mission statement is: Transforming managers into agile leaders of change and performance through neuroscience principles.

In doing so, we transform the manager's personal awareness and performance, emotion regulation and resilience, creativity, agility and coaching capability.

But why now? There are six key challenges I see facing business today.

1. Cognitive Overload and the lack of innovative problem solving (THINK)
2. Stress and illness related productivity loss (REGULATE)
3. Average performance and influencing levels (ENGAGE)
4. Keeping up with rapid and relentless change (ADAPT)
5. The need for a coaching approach to performance (DEVELOP)
6. Technical managers and their response to "soft skills" leadership training (A NEUROSCIENCE APPROACH)

Recognise a particular problem that your organisation is facing? Each of them links to a chapter of this book. Flip to the relevant chapter to find examples, a detailed break-down of the neuroscience involved, and solutions for your business.

1. Cognitive overload and the lack of innovative problem solving

We all need to do more with less. We are surrounded by 'always on' technology, out of control emails, and expectations to attend back-to-back meetings. Managers are so overloaded with commitments that they no longer feel a sense of control over their workload. They say "Emails rule my life!", "I can't get everything done!", "I no longer even prioritise!", "I can't think straight!", "I'm not spending any time on strategy, my day is completely reactive!", "We are not being creative or innovative in our approaches.", "We are falling behind!" Our brains are often multi-tasking, which risks the quality of our decisions and interactions. We are exhausted by mid-afternoon, and solve this by propping ourselves up with coffee, sugar fixes or stress hormones.

Do you relate to any of the above? You are amongst the thousands of corporate leaders struggling to feel comfortable with their own productivity and creativity. Now you have the opportunity to be one of the few to change it.

In our section THINK, we unpack our fast-paced, email avalanche, meeting crazy world. We look at ways to create time for prioritisation, reflection and strategy, to reduce meeting commitments, have more insights to problem solve, reduce multi-tasking, and gain back some level of control.

2. Stress and illness related productivity loss

There is a lot of stress and burnout in the workplace and rarely do I meet a manager that I am coaching or training that is not feeling overwhelmed at some level. They are incapable of dealing with the workload as described above. Change is challenging, and people are stressed about their ability to keep up.

How many people in your company are experiencing stress and burnout, or are overwhelmed with the workload and expectations? Claims for leave of absence due to stress is on the rise. In 2013, mental stress cost Australian businesses more than $10 billion, according to Safe Work Australia.[1]

Emotional Intelligence 360 reports and PRISM Brain Mapping reports often show that managers are not managing their stress well. In these cases, they are taking it out on others with frustration, aggression and impatience - in the worst instances leading to bullying and harassment claims. Alternatively, they are not managing stress internally (and don't show others that they're struggling). These people have negative internal dialogues, they catastrophise, are driven by fear, can't sleep well at night, and are heading straight towards break-downs or depression.

In our section on REGULATE we look at how to reset with a 30 second circuit breaker to get you back into a calm, controlled emotional state. We will build your resilience to be impacted less by the stress, and teach you to renew your mental capabilities throughout the day. You can be more innovative, effective, and in control, and this chapter shows you how to do it.

3. Average performance and influencing levels

In today's competitive, global market it is survival of the fittest at its toughest. Only those companies that are agile, retain and develop talent, have staff that are highly engaged, and are developing with a customer focus will survive.

Average performance is not sustainable in today's highly competitive, changing market. That seems pretty obvious. So why are we still seeing average performance? Here are some of the key reasons.

a. Low engagement

b. Poor teamwork and cohesiveness

c. Little real customer and sales focus

d. Infrequent coaching and performance conversations

e. Change is challenging

f. Lack of leadership

Technical teams today need to provide great internal and external customer service. IT departments, for example, are now expected to be much more customer-oriented and customer-centric, with both their internal and external stakeholders. Again, that's often not historically their natural strength. They know how to do their technical job, but they can be challenged by how to influence others, communicate effectively, build rapport, ask people questions and support people to help themselves.

Human resources professionals are another case in point. Increasingly, they are now expected to play a more strategic role in talent and performance. They want, and are expected to, hold a 'seat at the table'- a phrase we hear often that means to contribute to strategic decision making. What can we do to change this? We support HR teams by training them in coaching skills, strategic decision-making and influencing skills.

Overall, people in organisations need to influence more and direct less. These days, organisations are more like matrix systems, with flatter structures and less hierarchy. Leading in this structure is not a skill that all people naturally possess. However, these skills can be developed.

Performance in teamwork and effective collaboration is also another challenge for management groups. Because their roles have historically been siloed, there is high turn-over and restructure rates, and trust is low.

In ENGAGE we look at what it takes to build influence skills, performance, trust, collaboration, teamwork, motivation and high performance.

Drawing from my experience of 20 years in sales and sales management, and my training in the neuroscience of persuasion and influence, we've put together this chapter to help managers and individual contributors develop these skills. From newly formed teams to dysfunctional senior leadership teams, from finance teams in banks to sales teams in car companies, from customer service teams at universities to teams working for charities - all can benefit from the neuroscience of engagement, influence and performance.

4. Keeping up with rapid and relentless change

The constant sense of impending change leaves us feeling left behind. Organisational restructures, acquisitions, new technology, changing legislative requirements, and cost reduction programmes are no longer every few years. They are every few months. Managers who are often struggling themselves with the change have to inspire, influence and induct their team members into these new processes.

> *"The illiterate of the 21st century will not be those who cannot read and write, but those who cannot learn, unlearn, and relearn." Alvin Toffler*

Often managers don't really know enough about the details of the changes coming, but are still needing to communicate positively to their team about them.

New habits also need to be formed, like using a new CRM system or other technology. The brain is wired to save time and energy as well as automate as much as possible, so pre-existing habits are challenging to change.

Our chapter on ADAPT outlines how change occurs in the brain and how neuroplasticity occurs to support managers in their attempt to help others form new, high performance habits. It also looks at how to be an "Adaptive Leader" and navigate teams effectively through the challenging, disruptive change.

5. The need for a coaching approach to performance

The way companies focus on people development is also changing. Many companies adopt a method called 70-20-10 to development. Each number is a percentage: 10% is learnt in a classroom/workshop, 20% through mentoring and coaching and 70% through on-the-job activities.

The problem is that in most companies, the middle 20% -- the coaching and mentoring – is not done well. The purpose of the 20% is to ensure that team members implement new learnings from workshops as well as continuously improve their work processes. Why is this such a challenge? Many managers don't know how to coach; they haven't been shown. They also don't think they have the time nor do they understand the value of it. Many managers also believe that they are coaching! Yet really, they are merely explaining things, or showing people how to do things. This is not a strong way to develop potential, particularly of knowledge workers, and doesn't lend itself to the creation of innovative cultures.

The philosophy of 70-20-10 is a good start, but without great coaching, insights are not capitalised on and new performance habits are not formed. People don't practically, or sufficiently, apply some of their 70% on-the-job learning or their 10% workshop development.

Another challenge is how to move your company away from performance ratings. Performance appraisals and ratings are threatening for all involved. Deloitte, Disney, Australian Tax Office, Microsoft and many more local and international companies have either stopped using or are in the process of removing or reducing reliance on annual performance ratings. Their aim is to cut down the red tape, reduce the lost productivity and reduce the 'threat' state it creates.

Instead, they are increasing their coaching capability, a trend that has been gaining momentum over the last 15-20 years. This trend has rapidly ramped up in the past few years as part of the solution to performance ratings and the need to develop a high-performance culture.

Finally, the third challenge is how to move away from thinking that people's capabilities are fixed, and from judging based on performance, not potential.

> "Unless the manager or coach believes that people possess more capability than they are currently expressing, he will not be able to help them express it. He must think of his people in terms of their potential, not their performance."[2]

In our chapter on DEVELOP we provide managers with the key principles on how to coach using a brain-based methodology called GROW-WISE. More importantly though, managers learn at a neurological level how to have the greatest impact on performance through a growth mindset, insights, positive focus, and emotionally intelligent coaching.

6. Technical managers and their response to soft leadership training.

People get promoted up to management roles because they have demonstrated great capabilities in their previous roles. However, these previous roles are often dominated by quite different strengths to what's needed at the management level. Developing strengths in typically 'left brain' traits - being more analytical, concrete, logical, linear and sequential in reasoning – is what often gets people promoted.

But people are not quite so logical and linear. Leadership is far more about skills such as empathy, vision, communication, motivation and development. Yet often there has been little chance to develop these skills, or little attention placed on their development. Many managers have also had very little training in this area, or are resistant to it. Technical and professional managers often don't respond well to 'soft and fluffy' leadership training. This is a huge factor in the leadership gap.

Are you or have you experienced managers who are technically brilliant and yet are challenged by people leadership? This has become a greater challenge in the last 15-20 years, as more and more companies have rapidly grown in the technology, engineering and scientific fields.

Often when I start a training session with a group of technical managers, I am met with some body language that suggests resistance to the training (arms crossed, no smiles, leaning back). Generally, they are more interested in learning more about their technical area than to attend training on 'leadership' or 'people development' related topics.

Interestingly, once the managers are introduced to the anatomy of the brain and understand how decisions occur, and how our executive functions are impacted by emotion processing in the brain, their body language changes. They are open and engaged (smiles, talking, sitting forward).

This kind of training speaks a language of evidence and facts, rather than theory and speculation, and this appeals to the technical manager.

Over the years of training for various traditional leadership companies I have found that the programmes typically offer models of how to do things without the understanding of the reason the model works. This is not effective nor empowering! If you want managers to be engaged, it is helpful if they have an understanding of their own brain mechanics. Give them the tools to have more insights. That's the way we've motivated managers to 'engineer their own change and change in others.'

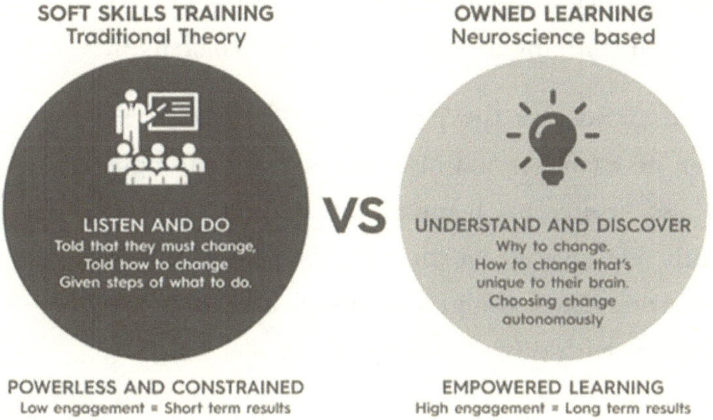

Source: Enhansen Performance

Once managers have a scientific understanding of how people work - how the brain works - it becomes easier for them to understand and navigate the intricacies of human behaviour. Rod, a senior manager from an engineering background in a Queensland

Government organisation, says there are three key things he's learnt about leading people through our training and coaching;

1. "It isn't easy!" But the neuroscience has made it much more comprehensible, and learning to coach effectively has supported the process.
2. "Value the talent of each individual." Gaining insight to a person's capability and talents only comes from having authentic and regular conversations. And this needs to be about the person, not just the tasks that need completing.
3. "It takes continuous effort to develop people". There is no silver bullet. You need to make reminders to shift your habits, for example that of telling people the answer instead of supporting their thinking to solving their own challenges.

Sounds all too hard? Rod says the pay-off and feedback he's receiving both from his manager and his staff is overwhelmingly positive and he's also seeing his team members' performance improve significantly. He says it's worth the effort. He's aiming to speak at an industry event for engineers and is keen to share more about his journey with others in his position.

Source: EnHansen Performance

The skills that are improved with our NeuroTREAD framework are:

THINK

- Self-awareness and Self-leadership
- Decision-making

- Understanding bias
- Productivity and mental performance
- Innovative problem solving
- Focus

REGULATE

- Stress management
- Resilience
- Emotional intelligence
- Cognitive and creative mental recharge
- Mindfulness

ENGAGE

- Teamwork
- Engagement
- Performance
- Influence
- Positive culture

ADAPT

- Agility
- Adaptive Leadership
- Habit formation
- Leading Change

DEVELOP

- Coaching
- Growth mindset
- Goal setting
- Performance conversations

- Feedback

> "We're more likely to need leaders who are good at facilitating new solutions than having all the answers. That is quite a different skill set from someone who is used to just getting more and more expert."[3]

The Neuroscience of Leadership

Neuroleadership is a term first coined by Dr David Rock in 2006. It is the field of neuroscience as applied to leadership. This book is not about all the detailed aspects of neuroscience, but about how integrated applied neuroscience relates to leadership and personal performance.

Why is neuroscience so relevant to leadership? The more we know about how the brain works, the more we can solve the challenges leaders face today, and the better outcomes we can get in our teams. What I'm sharing with you is based on my post-graduate studies in Neuroscience of Leadership with Middlesex University in the United Kingdom, my personal experience, my professional learning from working with top-tier clients in the past ten years, and from exposure to key neuroscientists that have worked in this space.

Technological advances that are changing brain science

Technological advances such as functional magnetic resonance images (fMRI) scans have made such progress in the last two decades. They've given us amazing insight into the way our brains work, enabling us to then use our brains to a greater level of potential.

The fMRIs measure blood flow. If you've ever had a look at a scan, you may have seen blue and red blotches on the brain images. Those blotches are showing increased and decreased blood flow.

Why is blood flow so important? Tracking blood flow has enabled neuroscientists to be able to see what parts of the brain are actively working, depending on the task or stimulus faced by the participant. Scientists observe which parts of the brain 'light up.' For example, when we show someone a scary face that causes them concern, the limbic system - the emotional part of the brain - lights up. It is getting greater blood flow. Likewise, when participants involved in the research are asked to make a decision, we see the part of the brain involved in decision-making 'light-up'. Researchers have been able to piece together what parts of the brain are involved in different activities by using different stimuli.

Electroencephalograms measure brain waves.

There's another way that scientists track brain activity. You may have heard of different types of brain waves such as theta, delta, alpha and beta. Electroencephalograms, or EEG's measure this electrical activity in the brain. They show a series of wavy lines that depict the waves that are present at the time of the reading. An EEG can help diagnose a number of conditions including epilepsy, sleep disorders, and brain tumours. It has also shown neuroscientists more about the different brainwaves involved in different activities, such as insight. We will be looking at this more in the chapter THINK.

Following such technological advances, research has shed light on five key areas that make up the field of the neuroscience of leadership. In brackets, you can see how each of these areas matches up with a focus from the NeuroTREAD framework - How to Think, Regulate, Engage, Adapt and Develop with the brain in mind.

- Decision-making and problem-solving (Think)
- Emotion regulation and resilience (Regulate)
- Engaging and collaborating with others (Engage)
- Adaptability, change and new habit formation (Adapt)
- Developing others (Develop)

A good proportion of the day for any manager or leader would be involved in dealing with these areas.

How the requirements of leadership have changed in the last 100 years.

Here is a quote from an article called 'The lives and times of the CEO' in the magazine Strategy & Business.

> 'Leadership has experienced an amazing evolution and the road ahead is going to be less and less predictable. It will require every ounce of flexibility, emotional intelligence, and creative thinking that executives possess.'[4]

Neuroscience sheds light on each of these areas: what it takes to be flexible and agile; how the brain changes even though it is resistant to change; how we can understand the neuroscience of emotion awareness, reasoning, influence and regulation; and how we can generate creative and innovative thinking through insight, diversity and empowerment.

That is a very different view of what CEOs and senior leaders needed if we compare it to 1914; 1964; and even 2014. In 1914 the priority was to cut turn-over rates in labour and raise productivity. The head of a company had absolute power, generally because he was the founder. This was the era of Henry Ford. By 1964 globalisation was becoming real, and companies were expanding to a whole host of different sectors. The CEO was no longer just managing a product they had created, but a complex executive suite.

Today's leadership needs have evolved again. Nowadays leadership involves:

- Flatter hierarchies
- Integrated technologies
- More women in senior and CEO roles
- Leading significant and regular change,
- Empathy
- Technological know-how

NeuroTREAD – Our program for applying Neuroscience to Leadership

There is barely an area involved in human performance that neuroscience can't shed light on today. Our NeuroTREAD framework aims to highlight the latest neuroscience in each of the areas that managers are involved in on a day to day basis.

TREAD stands for Think, Regulate, Engage, Adapt and Develop, with the brain in mind.

I developed NeuroTREAD as a framework to share the key neuroscience-based strategies I have learnt through my studies, my work with neuroscientists, my experience and my work with clients. In the past five years, over 7000 managers have been involved in learning insights from the NeuroTREAD program. The neuroscience of leadership is applicable across many different sectors. For example, I've delivered NeuroTREAD training to organisations from major banks and financial institutions to manufacturing companies, major telecommunications and technology service providers and various local, state and federal government organisations.

While it's a broad cross-section of companies, what is common to them is an innovative HR, learning and development (L&D) or talent manager, or a CEO who understands that a neuroscientific approach is more influential for their managers than relying solely on a traditional approach to leadership development. The groundswell and awareness has grown so rapidly in the last few years that many of these people have already been exposed to some of the research via the internet or presentations, and can immediately see the benefits of this approach even before we meet with them.

What we're seeing here is not a tiny trend. It is big wave of human understanding that has only just begun in the field of performance. This trend is gaining momentum now. It has gone past the early innovative stage, into the adopter's phase, and is rapidly heading towards the early majority. I called my framework NeuroTREAD because I believe that having science at the heart of leadership development adds real TRACTION to leadership development.

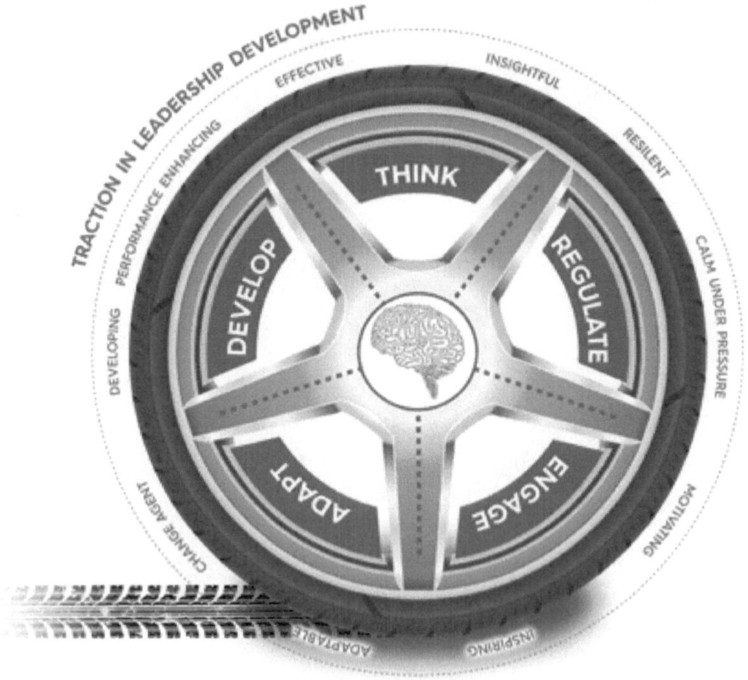

Source: Enhansen Performance

Imagine the difference between driving on a slippery road with bald tires, or driving on tires with new tread. Do you currently have performance tread for today's conditions? Do you have traction?

When people understand the mechanics of the brain and engineer their own change, with new 'tread' on their tyres or performance vehicles, it creates so much more ability to manoeuvre around the challenging terrain and deal with the ever-changing conditions managers face today.

Many managers are struggling. There is too much to do, with too few resources to do it, and always-on technology, endless meetings, flatter structures and global competition make it harder.

These are some of the things I hear regularly:

> 'My inbox rules my life and I can't get anything done!' (THINK)
>
> 'I don't have enough time to develop staff!' (DEVELOP)
>
> 'I'm always switched on and don't have any down-time anymore!' (THINK)
>
> 'I don't have time for exercise or to eat properly as my day starts on the phone at 7am and I'm not done with our international colleagues sometimes way into the night' (REGULATE)
>
> 'I'm stressed constantly and that makes it hard to manage effectively!' (REGULATE)
>
> 'My team are exhausted from all the constant change!' (ADAPT)
>
> "How can we keep being expected to do more with less?" (ADAPT)
>
> "I'm so used to solving people's problems, it's a habit that not easy to change!" (ADAPT)

> 'Our managers don't know how to have performance conversations!' (DEVELOP)
>
> 'I'm worried if I have performance conversations, I'll be pulled up for bullying or my staff will take stress leave!' (DEVELOP)
>
> 'We don't know how to get the managers to deal with their own performance issues!' (DEVELOP)
>
> 'My team expect me to have the answers and don't like thinking for themselves!' (DEVELOP)

Do we have to stay at this current level of capability? What is the impact on our organisations, and on us as leaders, if we don't address these challenges?

NeuroTREAD roadmap transforming Managers to agile Leaders of change and performance

If, as a manager, you want more innovative and strategic problem solving, greater resilience, higher engagement, more agile teams and higher performance, you need to develop your leadership skills in both self-leadership and leadership of others. Our NeuroTREAD framework summarises the shifts that you can make. It's not to leave behind management aspects but to engage in a good proportion of leadership attributes throughout your day. We've summarised the shifts we develop managers in during our programmes over 6-9 months. Many of these are discussed in this book throughout the NeuroTREAD framework. Accelerate your leadership with NeuroTREAD.

NeuroTREAD™ Roadmap
Transforming Managers to Agile Leaders of Change and Performance

	MANAGER	LEADER
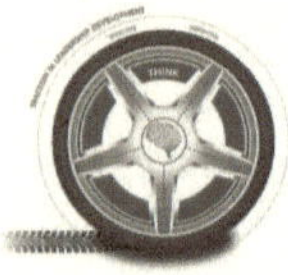 THINK	Manages by threat (have to do)	Leads with reward (want to do)
	Deliverables focused	Purpose and mission focused
	Consistent	Self-aware and agile
	Logic driven	Insight driven
	Operational	Strategic
	Detail oriented	Broad orientated
	Present road map	Future direction
	Multi-tasks	Focused
	Evaluates	Innovates
	Completes projects	Initiates projects
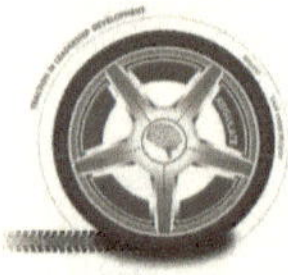 REGULATE	Cognitively intelligent	Emotionally intelligent
	Reactive/default response	Pro-active/intentional response
	Manages under pressure	Resilient under pressure
	Puts out fires	Avoids fires (back burn)
	Time management oriented	Energy creation oriented
	Works hard	Work smart
	Output commitment	Well-being commitment
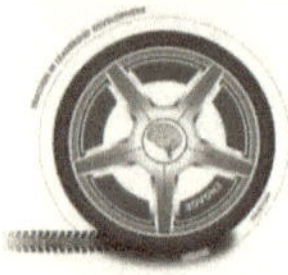 ENGAGE	Controls	Motivates
	Role based work asignment	Strength/passion based work alignment
	Manages team	Leads individual / Coaches team
	Task focused	People focused
	Siloed position strengths	Enterprise wide influence strengths
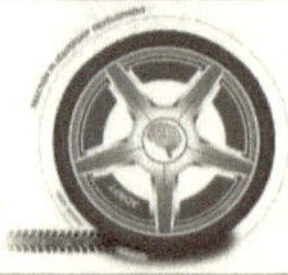 ADAPT	Maintains status quo	Leads change
	Solves technical challenges	Solves adaptive challenges
	Procedural	Flexible
	Fixed mindset	Growth mindset
	Describes performance expectations	Embeds new high performance habits
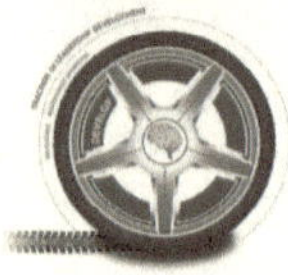 DEVELOP	Co-ordinates	Coaches
	Tells	Asks
	Solves problems	Generates Insight
	Provides solutions	Empowers others
	Delivers feedback	Illicits feedback
	Measures performance	Inspires Potential
	Directs	Influences

Source: Enhansen Performance

Summary

The need for, and availability of, a scientific approach to performance and leadership has never been stronger. With the constraints of rapid change, globalisation, increased competitive conditions, the need for growing technical specialist people managers, meeting higher expectations, influencing and developing people, and dealing with high levels of stress and burnout, it's clear that managers need support to lead teams to high and sustainable performance.

'TRACTION: The neuroscience of leadership and performance' is a summary of the key neuroscience-based principles and strategies derived from research that I have summarised into a framework called NeuroTREAD. It is about using a neuroscientific approach to Think, Regulate, Engage, Adapt and Develop with the brain in mind.

Reading this book will provide you with an understanding of how neuroscience can be applied to leadership, and with practical ways to apply it, starting today. What does that mean for you? Greater satisfaction in your day-to-day work life and better performance at work.

I hope you are inspired by this book to be the best leader and create the best leaders. By understanding more about human resilience, motivation, agility and performance we can meet the ever-changing, challenging conditions that we face in achieving personal and organisational success today!

Consider the following questions as you read this book

It's helpful to reflect on the following questions about your own leadership and performance, and that of others in your workplace, as you go through this book. You can see how you can apply these ideas in a practical way.

1. What are the key challenges faced by you, your managers, or your staff when it comes to performance and leadership?
2. What shifts do you or your managers need to make to provide greater leadership from the summary aspects above?
3. What are your skill gaps regarding leadership and performance?
4. What are you doing to build an innovative culture? How can you improve decision-making and problem solving to be more innovative to meet the future needs of your customers?
5. How are your change initiatives succeeding and what change do you have to lead in the coming years? Are your managers equipped to lead this? What is the current impact of change on your team or organisation?
6. How are decisions in your workplace made? Are they impacted by unconscious bias? How are your initiatives to lead diversity and inclusion going?
7. What is the impact of your performance ratings and appraisal systems and processes? Are they brain-friendly and performance enhancing?
8. How equipped are you or your managers at coaching for high performance and engagement? Can you afford to personally or organisationally not strive for peak performance?
9. Are you, your managers and your staff resilient? Are you or they experiencing stress and burnout? Is there constant pressure to do more with less?

10. Would you and your managers prefer a scientific evidence-based approach to performance and leadership than a 'soft' approach to these 'people skills'?
11. Are you and your managers prepared to recognise that change is going to continue to come at a rapid rate and you need to be equipped to build self-leadership strategies to have TRACTION to perform in these conditions?

PART ONE
THINK

CHAPTER ONE

Brain basics

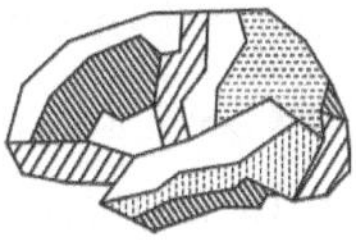

Let's have a look at some basics about brain structures and their role. Some of you might know a little bit about this and some of you may not, so I'm just going to start from the beginning to make sure we all are on the same page.

There are so many structures in the brain – hundreds – but we are only going to talk about a few. These are the ones that make a huge difference in everyday human life and that are most relevant to our understanding as leaders.

The first part is the prefrontal cortex (PFC), located at the front of the brain behind the forehead. The prefrontal cortex is responsible for our executive function, and it's known casually as our 'thinking' brain.

Here's what we include as executive functions:

- Decision making
- Planning
- Problem solving
- Logic

- Understanding
- Recall (taking from the long-term memory in to our working memory)
- Inhibition (stop ourselves from doing things)

The prefrontal cortex is the conscious part of our brain and our working memory. The prefrontal cortex is a busy part of the brain. But it's only 4% of the whole brain in terms of mass. We could also call the prefrontal cortex the 'hungry brain', because it consumes a significant amount of the glucose that we intake every day to function. It's very resource- and energy-inefficient compared to the rest of the brain. What a demanding part!

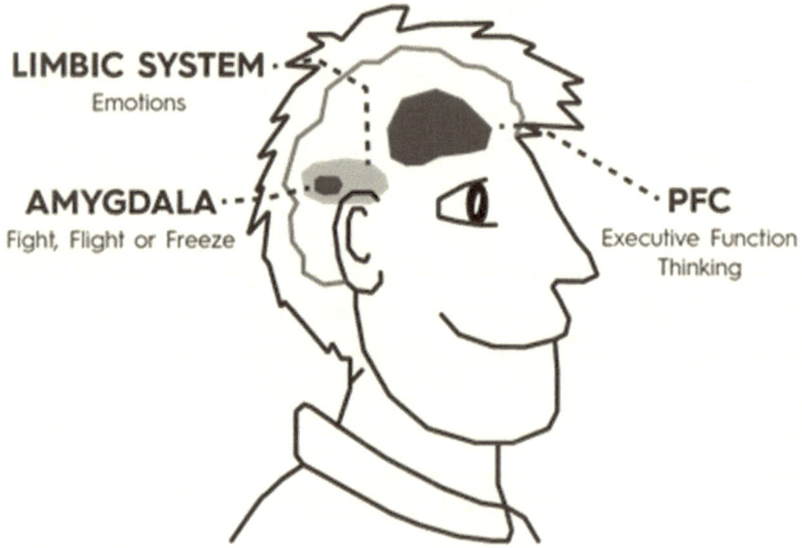

Source: Enhansen Performance

Amy Arnsten, who has studied the prefrontal cortex for over 25 years, describes it below:

> "The prefrontal cortex (PFC)—the most evolved brain region—subserves our highest-order cognitive abilities. However, it is also the brain region that is most sensitive to the detrimental effects of stress exposure. Even quite mild acute uncontrollable stress can cause a rapid and dramatic loss of prefrontal cognitive abilities, and more prolonged stress exposure causes architectural changes in prefrontal dendrites."[5]

What fuels the prefrontal cortex? Oxygen and glucose. These two elements are the fuel for the brain. And what brings the fuel to the prefrontal cortex and powers it? **Blood.** Blood brings the oxygen and the glucose to the brain and gives it the ability to function. It's filling up and recharging for every day as we sleep overnight.

When there is not enough blood flow, our prefrontal cortex doesn't work as well as it could. A client of mine calls it "sleepy brain after lunch" and says she doesn't get on with the proposals she has put aside till then because she can't think as clearly as in the mornings. She is concerned that she is missing a couple of hours of performance while this happens.

Let's look at a simple example of how to use this information about the brain to create a more effective workplace. We typically get to a point where our prefrontal cortex is depleted at about 3 o'clock in the afternoon. Although this is a generalisation, it's a pretty reasonable one. Up to 40% of every group I have ever trained experiences this afternoon dip sometime between 2-3pm. That is a great time to answer emails. It is not a great time to start a new project, because there is not much fuel left; our prefrontal cortex feels like it's running out of gas. We can feel tired, less creative, and experience more mental blockages.

This information has some clear implications for the way we approach our work day. Some neuroscientists say that we have four hours a day of optimal thinking and decision-making. Usually, that means we do our best work before lunch time, at which point things start to dip down. Our circadian rhythm also dips down in the afternoon. That's why a lot of European countries have a siesta – an after lunch nap – because we have that dip in the afternoon. But most of the world just pushes through that dip, often with a sweet treat, coffee or adrenalin, and it passes.

If our brain usually does our best thinking in the morning, it's worth considering what we are planning to complete for the day. How have we planned those activities? Are we using our thinking brain in the right way and at the best time? A lot of executives are starting to reorganise according to the functioning of the brain. They may avoid meetings in the morning. That is the ideal time for reflection, strategy, organisation, and prioritising. These types of work are taxing on our brain fuel, so we need to have a full tank. It seems for many people morning is their best time (usually around 70-80% of the workshop group), however for a few people the afternoon or evening is better. Young management teams generally have a broader mix and for many their brains aren't at their best until late morning or early afternoon.

Meetings stimulate blood flow. The simple process of interaction with other people helps spark us up. So, it makes great sense to move meetings and working with others to the afternoon. If you need to have a morning meeting, make them strategic and creative meetings. The afternoon is a great time for a work-in-progress meeting.

For those of you who have your best thinking in the afternoon or evening, are you arranging your day in the best way to capitalise on this?

The limbic system

Located more towards the middle part of the brain is the limbic system. It is responsible for processing our emotions. A key structure of the limbic system is the **amygdala**. The amygdala has a powerful role. It is responsible for our survival. How does it do that? It triggers our three Fs – our fight, flight or freeze response to threats.

The amygdala is a fascinating part of our brains. For example, there's an inverse relationship in between blood flow in the amygdala and in the prefrontal cortex, according to Matt Lieberman, Professor and Social Cognitive Neuroscience Lab Director at UCLA Department of Psychology, Psychiatry and Biobehavioral Sciences.

When we are in the fight-flight-freeze response, the blood flows to the heart and lungs and limbs. It drains away from the prefrontal cortex, and heads south. We need the blood in these areas so we can fight, run away, or stay very still.

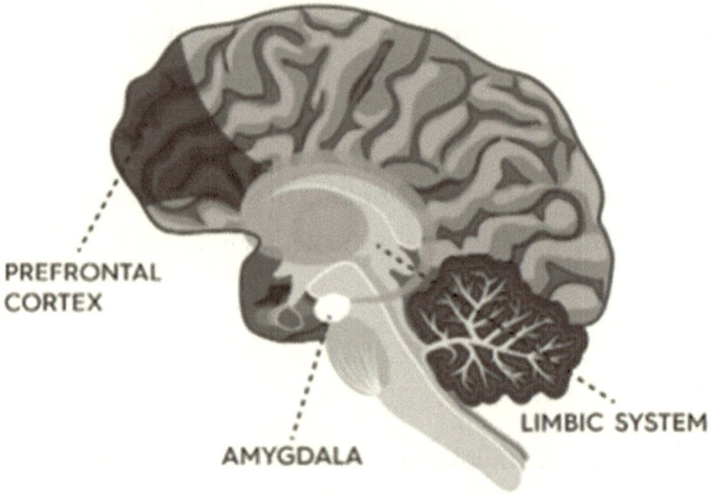

Source: Enhansen Performance

But there is more to it than that. If we need to respond quickly and automatically, we actually need to deactivate the prefrontal cortex. We wouldn't be here today if we used our thinking brain to work out what we should do when we come face to face with a predator. Hypothetically, if a bear walked into our office, and we were still using our prefrontal cortex to determine our next move, we'd be going: "Hmm let me have a think about that. I should introduce myself to the bear. Nah, probably it wouldn't be interested ..." And by that point we've already been attacked and killed by the bear. We are all here today because we have been designed so that we don't think that way when there is danger.

While the amygdala is responsible for our survival, it also can create havoc for us if we let it take over. There are a whole range of different responses to life-threatening situations. Some people would just freeze in the face of a disaster and won't save themselves at all. Other people would push everyone out of the way to get down the stairs in a fire and make sure they survive. It's not unlike a pilot having control of the plane wrestled from him by a hijacker. Without his consent, suddenly the plane takes a new course, unplanned and uncharted, with potentially disastrous results.

It is for this reason that unwanted amygdala interventions are known as an "amygdala hijack"!

Blood flow in the PFC and Amygdala

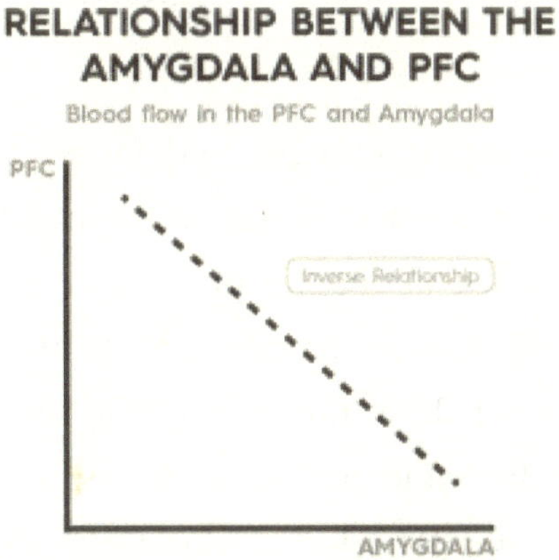

Source: Enhansen Performance

That's what happens to us we are under pressure, when we can't think straight. It happens regularly to some of us. But not all people are susceptible to their amygdala hijack, and not in the same way. Some people, particularly those in security and emergency response, have trained to respond with a coping strategy to the amygdala hijack. In a disaster situation, they have the presence of mind to respond in the way they've been trained, rather than the way their instincts would have them. Everybody responds to this fight-flight-freeze quite differently.

Interestingly, our life experience affects our response in a continuing way. The more stress you experience, the more your amygdala grows. It enlarges and makes more connections to the hippocampus (the long-term memory centre). People who have been traumatised and suffer post-traumatic stress disorders have enlarged amygdala's. Even more fascinatingly, our parents' response to stress can affect us even before we are born. The more you experience stress without coping strategies, the more your amygdala will grow.

I recently worked with an obstetrician who told me she has to deal with babies that become stuck in the birth canal. A colleague gave her some feedback about her physical response to this birthing crisis. "You look so worried when the babies are stuck," he said to her. "You can't show the mums that you are having a heart attack because the babies are stuck." To her credit, she took this feedback in and we did a lot of training together to help her to cope with her limbic system's response to calm the amygdala hijack. We talked through what she can do when she has an amygdala reaction. It's remarkable, but when she can show the mothers that she is calm at the moment of the crisis, it also helps the mothers stay calm. She has learnt to control her amygdala response and not let it get the best of her.

So, in a nutshell, we all deal with amygdala hijack very differently.

We will look at some strategies to use when your amygdala gets a bit jumpy further into this book.

The amygdala hijack experts

If you go into the army or military, you are trained for disasters. You are drilled again and again about what you need to do. Pilots are the same. They are trained for disaster. And yet, not every pilot could execute a successful emergency landing on the Hudson River, as Captain Chesley Sullenberger did with flight 1549 in 2009. So, we can see training can really make a difference for careers where people are dealing with life and death situations and need to have their wits about them. They must be able to calm their amygdala down, or have a relatively calm amygdala to begin with. And which part of the brain do we use to calm down and inhibit our amygdala? It's the ability of our prefrontal cortex.

There is a direct relationship between how well our prefrontal cortex is developed and how well we can control our amygdala. This is best demonstrated by a child or toddler who doesn't have a very developed prefrontal cortex. Having not yet learnt to regulate emotions, children often lose their minds if you simply take a toy away.

The toddler doesn't yet have the ability to say "Hang on, everything's going to be okay, maybe if I just wait for five minutes and share with my friend, I can get it back." Or a 13-year-boy, who rang his mum (my colleague) in hysterics because he couldn't get his phone charger to work and he only had 2% battery left. When she asked him "On a scale of 1 to 10, with 10 being death, where are we?" his answer was "We are at a nine." His prefrontal cortex was not developed enough to deal with that amygdala hijack.

The prefrontal cortex isn't fully developed in men until mid-twenties, and in women until early-twenties. That's why a teenager is just one big walking amygdala and nothing makes sense to their logical brain because they are so emotional. That's why young men in their late teens and early 20s, who already have a lot of testosterone and adrenaline surging in their system, are at risk when they have a few drinks. The alcohol reduces the function of the prefrontal cortex, which is only partially developed anyway. Picture the bouncer of a nightclub saying to a 19 year old that has had a few drinks, "No, you're not coming in here, mate, you look like you've had a few too many drinks". Their amygdala gets aroused with little control capability and he may king hit the bouncer. We have all heard of disastrous outcomes as a result. People can go from just being a normal guy to being a drunken physically violent "thug". We don't get better at thinking in our threat state. The only thing we get better at when we are in a threat state is motor function, so we can become stronger and faster, and we can hit a lot harder.

CHAPTER TWO

The amygdala in business

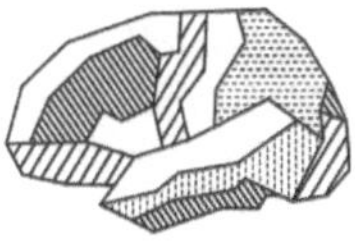

Take a typical manager of factory employees, say 50 to 100 years ago. If they called out one of their workers and said "Hey, let's go a bit faster, otherwise don't come back tomorrow", the employee would go into a threat state and work faster. The resulting increase in output would have the manager think, "I'm a good manager. I didn't need my workers to think; I just needed them to do what they are doing faster, faster, faster". But today, we are now mainly managing knowledge workers. Unfortunately, as soon as the knowledge worker gets into the threat state, they are less capable. They can't think. For example, if I say to a thought worker "If you don't come up with the solution to the problem this afternoon, then don't come back tomorrow", they have got little chance of coming up with the most innovative way to solve the problem. As knowledge workers, we need the prefrontal cortex to be in a reward state, not a threat state, to be effective.

Threat and reward

Have a guess how often your brain scans the environment for danger, threat or reward. It's an incredible five times per second!

This understanding is from Integrative Neuroscientist Dr Evian Gordon's work. He found that the brain's organising principle is to minimise danger and maximise reward. This occurs largely unconsciously and extremely fast. It is much faster than the conscious prefrontal cortex conscious part of our brain.

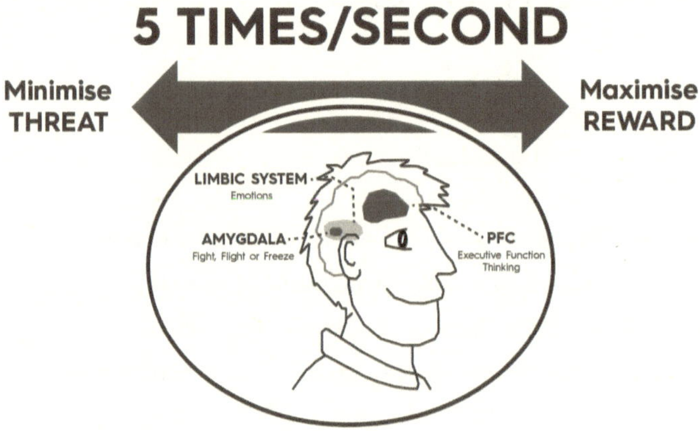

Source: Enhansen Performance

All negative emotions put us into a threat state. Frustration, anger, nervousness, worry, concern, fear, impatience. If we are in a threat state, neuroscientists have found our peripheral vision narrows, we become more risk averse, have less insights, feel less connected and we are problems focussed.

The good news is that all positive emotions put us in a reward state. Calm, happiness, interest, curiosity, gratitude, appreciation, excitement. If you are experiencing positive emotions, you are in a reward state. When we are in the reward state, we experience a broad focus, we are open to risk, we have more insights, we feel more connected, and are more solutions focussed. In business today, in order to get the best of ourselves and everybody else, we need to be in a reward state.

We deal with negative stressors quite differently and it is how we view these stressors that can make the biggest difference. If we see a stressor as a "challenge" instead of a "threat", then we can feel excited, energised and even confident in our ability to deal with it. Our body organises for oxygenated blood flow to go to our brain and body. This is how we "rise to the challenge" or can perform under tight deadlines.

It seems to be a fine line for many where the stress is viewed positively versus negatively, and we have to understand ourselves and others well to determine this. We also can practise positive reappraisal regularly when faced with a stress to see it as a positive challenge to gain the benefit from the stress. We will discuss this further in the "Regulate" section.

Threat and reward has also been described as an avoidance or approach state.

Researchers have found that the "Approach motivation tends to be related to activation of the left hemisphere, where avoidance motivation tends to be related to activation of the right hemisphere. Approach motivation seems to coincide with activation of the medial prefrontal cortex as well as the nucleus accumbens.[6] Avoidance motivation seems to coincide with activation of the amygdala and anterior cingulate cortex".[7]

The bear and the owl

There are no bears coming for us nowadays. Having said that, it's still pretty threatening out there. It's not easy, would you agree?

Many organizations have people feeling quite threatened in their everyday jobs. They are expected to do more with less. We have less resources to do more things. There is always change. There is constant technological update, there is constant process update or there is a threat of an acquisition or merger. You may also have a new manager this week, a new IT or customers service system to navigate, you're going to have an open desk policy next week. Do this, do that, differently. And your brain is going "Give me a break, this is not easy!"

For us as leaders, a key role is being able to help people to create a reward state amongst the threat. The first step for leaders, if we are going to help others, is to recognize when we feel in threat state, and learn how to get ourselves out of it. What kind of times may put us under threat? When we feel ourselves under too much pressure, or when our senior management has told us we need to perform more, then we are in a threat state.

Friedman and Foerster conducted a curious experiment in which they put a large number of undergraduates in a room to work on a mouse maze.[8] They divided the room in half. In the experiment, the participants worked on a mouse maze that depicted either a piece of "cheese" for the mouse as it exited the maze, or an "owl" as it exited the maze. Following this stage, all of the mouse mazes were collected and all of the participants were given a visual problem-solving task which involved insight.

Which side of the room solved more perceptual problems? By how much do you think?

The people completing the cheese maze solved more and by approximately 50%.

They found that the approach maze completion (cheese) was indeed associated with attentional broadening on this task, whereas avoidance maze completion (owl) engendered relatively narrow attention, a tendency to focus on the "trees" rather than the "forest". "Critically, this manipulation showed no reliable influence on self-reported emotional feelings or mood, supporting the contention that they operate merely as implicit affective cues". In other words, people were not aware they were in a threat state. They didn't 'feel' stressed, yet nonetheless the owl had narrowed their focus and reduced their ability to solve these perceptual, creative problems.

Friedman and Foerster had wanted to see if even a small threat can reduce problem solving capabilities significantly. To think that these participants with the cheese on the maze beat the others by 50% just because they had a picture of an owl on the page! We are not mice! The difference between cheese and owls is hardly relevant to a human. Owls don't even hurt humans! And, it was just a picture on a piece of paper. So why? Why does a stimulus like this still have an effect? Because a lot of what goes on in our brain is unconscious. We don't even have to be consciously aware that we are in a threat state for it to reduce our problem-solving capabilities.

How is this relevant to us as leaders? What should we do to help get our team members out of that threat state and into a reward state? We should remember that a threat doesn't have to be a bear-type threat to inhibit our performance. It can be very small. For example, I am a manager and I say to one of my staff: "Can I see you in my office in five minutes please?" Uh-oh. Immediately she thinks, "Oh no, what have I done?" She is already in a threat state. She is unlikely to tell me about all the concerns or problems she is having because she is waiting to hear what am I going to pounce on her for, what has she done wrong, what she missed. Alternatively, I could come in to the office and say: "Hi, I just wanted to pick up on the project from last week and get your input for a meeting I am attending, do you have 10 minutes this morning?" In this scenario, she is more likely to respond by saying, "Sure, happy to update you, all pretty good except we do need to be aware of one challenge". As leaders, we've got to recognize that simple management questions, or telling someone what to do rather than asking them, is enough to create a threat state.

Ask, don't tell

Knowledge workers are motivated by autonomy. That is one of the key reasons that coaching - asking not telling – is making a huge inroad in organisations now. We take away that autonomy all too often. Imagine if someone is stuck with a dilemma, and we say: "Tony, you know what you need to do, you need to go and see Michael, and please make sure you tell Michael the following." If that's not what Tony wants to do to solve the problem, then he is already in a threat state. You are telling him what to do, and there is immense social pressure on him to do it. This is clearly not the most expansive mindset for both parties to be in. Yet that is exactly what most managers do. We tell, we do not ask.

Instead, we need to empower people to do things on their own. You will always need to advise someone when they begin a role to help them understand how things should be done. Once they get the gist of a role, give them the space to really own it. This depends on the level of seniority and knowledge of the role, but the reason people often request job descriptions is so they know what they should be doing and where their focus should be. They want to be able to do it on their own!

This is where the situational coaching comes in. We need to give people some certainties, so people feel that they know what they are supposed to be doing. Once we've done that, we need to ask them "What do you think?" We need to create an environment where they can put their own ideas into solutions, and that's where the coaching comes into it. We will take a more detailed look at how to coach someone in our chapter on DEVELOP.

Summary

The brain determines non-consciously whether a stimulus or event is a threat or a reward approximately five times a second. Even a small threat can impact our cognitive and creative problem-solving capabilities significantly and reduce our desire to connect with others.

If managers are not conscious of how they are communicating, both verbally and through tone and body language, they can easily throw their team members into a threat state, thus reducing their ability to be effective.

When managers take a coaching approach to developing team members - by asking more than telling - they are supporting change in a non-threatening way and providing much more autonomy to their team member. This is more likely to create a reward state, lead to more insights and innovative solutions, and greater performance over time.

Consider the following questions

Given how sensitive we are to "threat" and "reward", and how it impacts our abilities to solve problems and be connected to others, what can we do as managers to create the right environment?

How do we reduce threat?

How do we increase reward?

Which of these are you doing well?

Which could be improved on?

What are other things that you could try or be more conscious of?

Examples of the above:

Reduce threat: increase communication, clarify expectations, role clarity, reasonable deadlines

Increase reward: recognition, fun environment, brain-breaks/ downtime, interesting projects, visually enjoyable workplace.

CHAPTER THREE

Conscious and non-conscious decision making

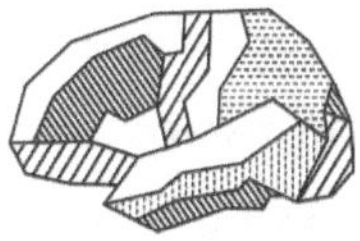

The prefrontal cortex – our conscious brain – is very small, deliberate and very limited in processing capacity. Meanwhile the non-conscious is fast and automatic.

> "Non-conscious brain processes have the capacity of encoding vast amounts of information relative to complex events of the physical world through multiple interdependent sensory channels at any given moment of time. Conscious processing, on the other hand, is extremely limited in capacity, which explains why most of our knowledge of the world is generated outside consciousness." [9]

Winner of the Nobel Prize Daniel Kahneman, in his book Thinking Fast, Thinking Slow, refers to this by describing our non-conscious as System 1.[10] This is described as "fast, intuitive, associative, metaphorical, automatic, impressionistic, and it can't be switched off".[11] System 2 thinking, done by our prefrontal cortex and conscious brain, is relatively slow and deliberate.

As managers, we need to be aware of the capacity of the non-conscious brain. We need to know when to override it, to calm it down and to use the prefrontal cortex to get ourselves out of sticky or automatic response situations.

A great thing about coaching effectively is that it also taps in to non-conscious processing. If we ask our staff members great reflective questions that are not readily available in their conscious thinking, we are tapping into the non-conscious. We are tapping into what is not known, and we are helping this person to have insights.

The insightful brain

Wag Dodge was a parachute smoke jumper leading a team of smokejumpers in 1949 in Montana on the hottest day on record. They were responding to a fire that had taken off in the Man Gulch region. Wag and his men landed on the steep, dry, grassy highlands to put out a small fire. Shortly after the wind changed direction and the men found themselves being chased up the steep hill by a raging fire, two hundred feet tall. Wag knew he could not outrun the fire as it had become too fast on the steep hill, but he knew of no procedural alternative. He screamed to his men to stop running, but nobody stopped. Dodge was telling the men to stand still.

In a desperate bid to save his life, Wag had a creative thought. He lit the grass in front of him, wet a handkerchief with some water from his water bottle and put this over his mouth and nose, and lay down in the smouldering embers. He waited, terrified, while the fire passed over him. Wag did this and was one of only two men out of thirteen to survive that day. Unfortunately, the panic his men felt narrowed their thoughts and senses, and they weren't able to see a solution. Wag Dodge, on the other hand, experienced an "insight" and it saved his life. Wag's fire escape is now a standard firefighting technique.[12]

In today's business world, most of us are lucky enough to not be facing raging fires. However, we are under enormous pressure to perform to deadlines under ever-changing conditions. These still create threat responses. Being able to remain calm under pressure is understood to be a positive leadership trait. On top of this, the ability to stay calm allows us to come up with innovative solutions to complex problems with no known previous experience. The knowledge about how to have "insights", and the brain-state required for insights, can help managers in these times of pressure to make more effective decisions.

Insights come from the non-conscious part of our brain; we become "suddenly" aware of them in our conscious brain. To harness the unconscious brain when trying to solve complex problems, we sometimes need to say to our conscious brain, "Leave it! Let the rest of my brain sort this out, as it's way more capable." When we get stuck, it's our little prefrontal cortex, which is slow at processing, that is not managing the complexity.

We can say "OK, I don't know the answer right now, but I will sleep on it or come back to it in an hour".

When we let the non-conscious work out problems, we sometimes get even better answers. The prefrontal cortex (conscious) shuts down at night but your non-conscious brain does not. It keeps going all day, every day. It will often sort out these big challenging problems for you that will come to you as an insight. We will take a detailed look at insight in the coming pages.

The right mix gets us in the zone

The prefrontal cortex is extremely fussy. What do I mean by 'fussy'? I mean that the prefrontal cortex needs exactly the right chemical mix to put us in either the 'feel good' mood or the 'feel bad' mood. There are many neurochemicals in our brain, but there are about 10 that do a lot of the work. They are:

Acetylcholine
Dopamine
Serotonin
Norepinephrine
Epinephrine
GABA
Glutamate
Histamine
Nitric oxide
Glycine

The prefrontal cortex needs just the right mix of neurochemicals for peak performance. That's when you are in the zone, when you are in a "flow" state. You have the perfect neurochemical mix for you, and that comes about from having just the right amount of challenge and just the right amount of skill.

This mix varies from person to person. If I want to get the very best out of Ben, I need to know what state he needs to be in mentally to get the best out of him. For some people that might mean saying, "Ben, don't worry. It's okay. Everything is going to be okay." But for other people, it might be best to say, "It's not enough. I need you to be up here, and you are nowhere near. But I think you can get here. Can you please jump a bit higher?" Some people we need to manage one way, and for others we need to manage another way, to encourage the greatest neurochemical mix for their peak performance.

Some people need more stretching and challenging; others need to feel more comfortable to be at their peak performance. When we have a team full of people, we need to get a feel for where they operate at their peak.

John is an accomplished sales person and enjoys the thrill of the biggest challenges. His best moments are in selling to large international 5-star resorts, clients that are considered a long-shot, but the deals are big and the pay-off is good. John's manager needs to ensure his territory and opportunities include these bigger clients. In an acquisition and restructure, John was instead handed a territory of a whole lot of already existing small hotels, and was asked to grow this territory. There were no big deals or negotiations, instead there was a lot more administration. The people he was dealing with were not as sophisticated when it came to the use of this technology, and didn't have the budget to upgrade.

This role was beneath John's capability. He was frustrated, disappointed, and felt undervalued – which resulted in low engagement and motivation, and subsequently poor results. John ended up on extended stress leave, costing the company productivity and money, and impacting John's health. This was as a result of him being given a territory that, from one perspective, should have been easier and less stressful for John. However, the demands of his manager and the lower level of challenge impacted his performance by underutilising his talents. John has now left this company and works for a competitor that recognises his talents. He is once again on the hunt for the challenging, large opportunities in the market, pitted against the company that didn't have the foresight or management capability to utilise him in the best way.

John's manager needs to understand that the neurochemical make-up and reaction to stimulus and activities is different for different people. To get the best from each of the individuals we manage you need to consider this, and adjust what you can to help people perform at their best.

On the left side of the curve, people are not experiencing enough arousal stress. Where people are under-stimulated, tired, or bored, they are not performing at their peak. Just before the top of the curve is the place familiarly known as your comfort zone. Some people are happy operating here, while others will want the constant stimulation to be aiming to be at peak performance. Leaders could raise the challenge by lifting expectations,

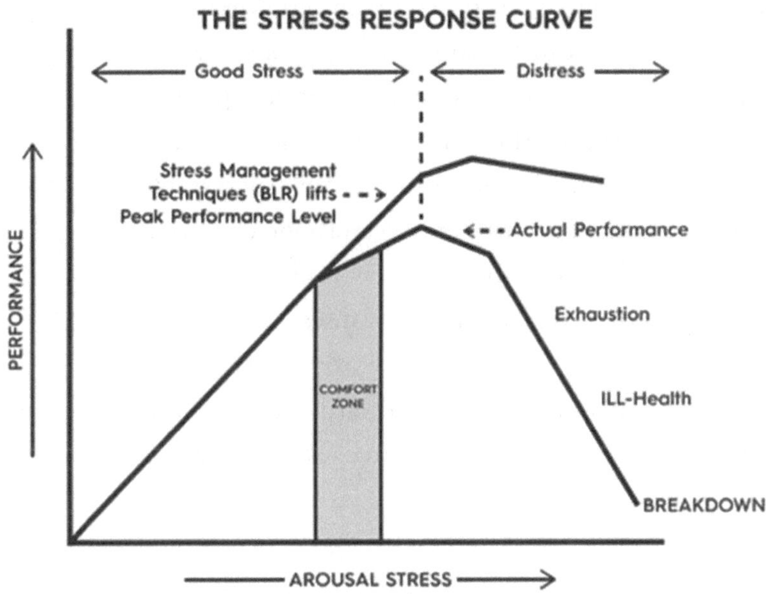

Source: Enhansen Performance

tightening deadlines, or asking them what would make the project more interesting and stimulating.

The aim is to have everyone in your team operating at their peak mental performance. But each person is different, so understanding that and discovering more about your team members can help you achieve this.

When we experience too much input (arousal), such as on the right side of the diagram above, there can be a sudden drop-off in performance. We experience black-and-white thinking; we are in distress, we are not organised, we are less connected to others, we are challenged by setting priorities and managing time; and we experience feelings of constant low-level panic and guilt.

In this over-arousal state, your brain processes things differently. Your brain takes the most automatic and easiest response. When we experience a state of fear or anxiety regularly, it changes the way your brain perceives the world and, over time, it can cause physical changes in the brain. Your attention and behaviour are then driven by threat-avoidance. This can become a vicious cycle where your brain perceives more threats in the environment – even if they are not there – which in turn causes more stress. Leaders should recognise this and create environments which encourage and support people (provide reward amongst the threat) to get them to their optimal dopamine level where the PFC functions at its peak.[13]

Tell your prefrontal cortex what it wants to hear

Although our prefrontal cortex is a fussy place, we can manage and control our own neurochemical mix much better than we think. For example, if we walk around criticising ourselves and saying to ourselves "I stuffed up" and "I can't do this", then we put ourselves in a threat state. We will not be in the best state to solve problems or make decisions. A big part of leadership is knowing which state we're in and what can we do to change it. And quickly! This makes us more resilient. For example, we may be tight to make a deadline on a project or a proposal, and then suddenly we have a staff issue we need to deal with urgently. This can easily throw us into a threat state, as we feel the pressure to complete two (or sometimes more than two) things at the same time, both reasonably urgent. Being aware of the impact of this and regulating our stress response could mean the difference between resolving the staff issue in a timely, creative and supporting way, or not.

We can manage the threats that are continuously coming at us if we build our resilience. It's about recharging our prefrontal cortex when it's running out of gas. We can take a break, eat a little nourishing food, have a stimulating talk with one or more people. We'll look at these options fully in the next chapter.

If it's so easy, why then don't we take sensible action? Why do we work through our exhaustion, and eat rubbish? Because it's our prefrontal cortex that houses our ability to inhibit, our ability to stop ourselves from doing things! In the morning, when we wake up and we have a fresh prefrontal cortex, that's when we might say that we are not going to eat any unhealthly food and we are going to do some exercise, we're not going to have any wine or beer this evening and we're not going to eat rubbish at 3pm in the afternoon. But by 3pm, following the stress of the day and the amount we have already inhibited, our prefrontal cortex has run out of energy to hold us to our previous decisions. We get to the point where we say "Forget that!" and end up eating an unhealthly choice, not getting out for some exercise, and finishing our day with a few beers or glasses of wine.

It is important to recognise that we do have good intentions. Our PFC has good control over our behaviour to inhibit in the morning when our brain is fresh. But as the day wears on, some people feel they lose the ability to inhibit their emotions and behaviour. That's why our family sometimes get the worse of us:

because we've been inhibiting all day long, stopping ourselves from saying "Come on, I've explained that already!" a few times. When somebody at home says something that annoys us in the evening, we often lash out and say what we think, without considering how to say it diplomatically.

Amy Arnsten has described the PFC to be similar to Goldilocks. Why do you think your prefrontal cortex has been described this way? Well, Goldilocks was pretty fussy! She wanted her porridge not to hot and not too cold, and the chair not too big or too small, and the bed not too hard or too soft, but everything "Just right". Our PFC wants everything to be just right to be at optimal performance. We need the neurochemical mix just right - not too happy, not too sad - just right. It's very fussy. But we can control it much more than we think!

Summary

It's worth knowing about two very useful structures in the brain. The first is the prefrontal cortex, which is responsible for our executive functions such as understanding, recalling, deciding, inhibiting, planning, and recalling. The second is the amygdala, a key structure in the limbic system that orchestrates our fight, flight, and freeze response to a perceived threat.

There is an inverse relationship between blood flow in the prefrontal cortex and the amygdala, which means that when we are experiencing a threat, we can't think straight.

CHAPTER FOUR

Insight

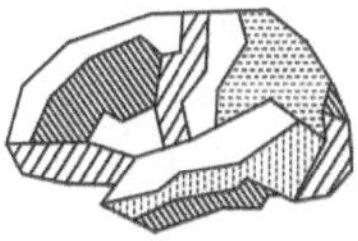

Let's take deeper look at insight. We've discussed the idea of insight a little bit. But what is an insight? Why are they important and how do they occur in the brain? What conditions are required to have insights? Can we make them happen more often?

The formal definition of insight is "a sudden realisation of a complicated situation" and the casual definition is an "aha or light-bulb moment".

Why are insights important? They are the seeds of creativity, problem solving, empowerment, and motivation. Insights are really powerful. They are absolutely amazing.

The prefrontal cortex does the logical problem solving: 2+2=4. Or, if I go here, that will mean X. But the non-conscious brain does much more. It's called "semantic-processing". What that means is that it's working all over the place. There are many different roads (neural pathways and connections) coming together from all directions at the same time. The non-conscious brain is taking in all this information and using it for its processing. This helps us with the more complicated understandings and decisions.

> "Brain activity fluctuates prior to each new problem, during a resting "preparatory period". Different patterns of activity occur prior to problems that people solve with insight versus prior to problems they solve more analytically. In the prep period before getting problems subsequently solved with insight, people have greater activity in the anterior cingulate cortex, a midline frontal area associated with cognitive control, and in bilateral temporal areas associated with semantic processing".[14]

By contrast, our prefrontal cortex is much more linear, and simplistic, and can only effectively hold a few things in mind at once to solve a problem. I was shocked when I discovered that our prefrontal cortex is this simple, and that all the complex thinking we do is going on behind the scenes. By becoming more aware of what goes on in our non-conscious processing, we can harness its capacity more effectively. As mentioned in the earlier chapters, it is possible to intentionally use our non-conscious processing to find us solutions. We can do this much more frequently if we truly understand what is going on inside our heads.

Why we love insights

From a neurochemical perspective, something very positive happens when we have an insight. We get a hit of dopamine. Dopamine has the same effect in the brain as a hit of cocaine. Dopamine is the feel-good neurochemical, and is so important for our daily functioning.

One of the current missed opportunities that we see in businesses is when someone comes to a manager with a problem, and the manager provides a solution. They say "You know what you need to do? Do x, y, z." Who gets the dopamine hit, do you think? The manager does. They are after that instant gratification of solving the problem, they often get thanked, and they feel good about helping. It is much more natural; it is our default to solve somebody's problem, get a dopamine hit ourselves, and send them on their way. Because we've done it quickly, efficiently, we get the boost of status because we've been able to help somebody else.

The problem is that the other person misses out. They don't get that same sort of dopamine hit as the manager. What if the manager helped someone to come up with the answer, instead of just giving it? Could they both effectively get the dopamine hit? The answer is yes. The staff member gets a hit when they come up with an answer. And the manager gets the dopamine hit that says, "I just helped someone get an insight." It is delayed gratification, but when you look at someone and think "I've facilitated somebody's improved thinking" – that's worth having a dopamine hit over.

There is a second crucial part to this. Dopamine hits that are associated with an insight pass quickly. You have that insight – "Aha yes, I got it!" – and then it goes. To help the person we are supporting to stay excited and energised, we have to get them to actively do something about it right there and then. When we have an insight, or when someone we are working with has an insight, we need to take the moment and say, "Great, what an excellent idea! What are you going to do about it?" "What action can you take now?"

How often do you see managers do that? What do we usually see instead? Someone has an insight, but because it's not the manager's insight, the manager just goes "Oh okay, I guess you could do that." When we see energy in somebody, when we see that they are onto a good thing, we need to recognise it and say "Well, that looks pretty energising! What can you do to act on it?"

Capturing the idea on paper is an effective first step. Outside of work, many people have insights around 2am-3am in the morning if they wake. When this happens, we need to write it down, because we know if we wait until we wake up in the morning, we are going to forget it.

Effective coaches tap into the energy of insights. They look for opportunities that allow people to have their own insights, and then capitalise on them. The best way to develop the people you are leading is through a series of insights, day after day after day.

Insightful times

When do we have our best insights? After asking thousands of people this question in the last few years, the following have stood out as the most popular places to have insights.

1. Shower (by far the number one)
2. In bed (either going to sleep or middle of the night)
3. Driving

4. Exercise

5. On the toilet

I usually turn this into a game when I have a room of people, and give them seven guesses to correctly guess the top five places that people have insights. Every group, even when there are 250 people in the room, all come up with the top five within seven guesses.

What do these top five places all have in common? People describe themselves as being relaxed - in what we call a quiet brain state – when they are in these places.

In these situations, our prefrontal cortex is quiet or calm. We all have such busy brains these days! Due to technology, we are often working our brains in a 'switched on' mode from the second we wake up in the morning to the time we go to sleep.

I'll describe what an insight looks like in the brain very simplistically. Imagine that your hands are a neuron with the cell nucleus (the palm) and the dendrites/axons (the fingers). Open your hands in front of you with the fingers of one hand almost touching some of the fingers of the other hand. The ends of your axon need to come close to the dendrites of other neurons. But they don't touch. They connect at what is called the synapse, and a synapse is a space, so it's not a physical connection. This space is where the neurochemicals jump from one axon to another.

Now, while our neurons are busy talking, there might be another neural pathway or connection over to one side that's a bit weaker.

Think of it as the distance between two fingers further away from each other. It's not quite as connected. As long as I'm talking and thinking about what I've got to do with my work, my kids, how many emails I have, I can't hear this weak connection. But when I eventually say "Be quiet, let's go for a walk, take a deep breath, relax, let's go to the gym", then I can actually hear that weak connection. Mark Jung-Beeman, an expert in the neuroscience of insights, states that "variables that improve the ability to detect weak associations may improve insight solving."[15]

How do insights occur?

Neuroscientists have researched to understand how the brain produces insights, and how this type of problem-solving differs from the more linear, logical problem-solving that occurs in the prefrontal cortex.

Research suggests that people often find solutions to challenges at an unconscious level, and the right cerebral hemisphere (RH) appears to be involved. The following is an excerpt from the article The Aha! Moment: The Neural Basis of Solving Problems with Insight, explaining a series of experiments used to test for insights.

> "To test this hypothesis, Jung-Beeman et al. mapped both the location and electrical signature of neural activity using functional magnetic resonance imaging (fMRI) and the electroencephalogram (EEG). In the first experiment, thirteen people were given three words (pine, crab, sauce) and asked to

think of one word that would form a compound word or phrase for each of the words (can you figure it out?). Neural activity was mapped with fMRI while the participants were given 124 similar word problems—which can be solved quickly with or without insight, and evoke a distinct Aha! moment about half the time they're solved. Subjects pressed a button to indicate whether they had solved the problem using insight, which they had been told leads to an Aha! experience characterized by suddenness and obviousness.

While several cortical regions showed about the same heightened activity for both insight and non-insight derived solutions, only the aSTG in the RH showed a robust insight effect. Given that neural activity in this area also increased when subjects first encountered the problem (perhaps reflecting unconscious processing), the authors conclude that the increase does not simply reflect the emotional jolt associated with insight.[16]

In a second experiment, 19 new participants engaged in the same type of problem-solving tasks as the first group while their brain waves were measured with an EEG.The researchers then analysed the EEG recordings to look for differences between insight and non-insight solutions in brain wave activity. The researchers found that 0.3 seconds before the subjects indicated solutions achieved through insight, there was a burst of neural activity of one particular type: high-frequency (gamma band) activity that is often thought to reflect complex cognitive processing. This activity was also mapped to the aSTG of the RH, providing compelling convergence across experiments and methods.

Problem-solving involves a complex cortical network to encode, retrieve, and evaluate information, but these results show that solving verbal problems with insight requires at least one additional component. Further, the fact that the effect occurred in RH aSTG suggests what that process may be: integration of distantly related information. Distinct neural processes, the authors conclude, underlie the sudden flash of insight that allows people to "see connections that previously eluded them."

How to have more insights!

Following Mark-Jung Beeman's work on insights, author and thought leader Dr David Rock summarised the research in an article called "The Aha Moment."[17]

Dr Rock summarised that four states increased the likelihood of an insight. We studied these during the post-graduate studies I completed through Middlesex University and they have been helpful for my coaching clients, as well as me personally, in improving problems. These four states were generalised as:

1. A quiet brain – Alpha brain waves – through closed eyes, exercise, deep breathing, relaxation, gardening, before sleep, and in the middle of sleep.
2. Not focussing directly on the problem.
3. Looking inward.
4. Being in a reward state rather than a threat state.

Anything you can do to experience these four states will make a huge difference to you in terms of having more insights. We are going to have a more detailed look at the above in order to understand these conditions required for insights.

So how do we get into these states? We have a convenient tool called the 5 R's of Insight – Recognise, Relax, Reflect, Remove and Reward.

The 5 R's of Insight!

Recognise

It is useful to firstly recognise that not all problems are created equal! Some problems are more suited to being solved in the PFC with a logical, sequential, and limited amount of data. Others, perhaps more complex, need some time for the brain's 100 billion neurons to have the opportunity to mull it over a little more. It is important to "recognise" when our brain is either too full with other competing needs to give adequate attention to a challenge, or if the problem has various inputs and is complex. In these cases, sometimes giving a little more time can help us see the solutions in a new way via an insight, a solution that simply wouldn't have occurred to us otherwise.

When I can't work something out I assess – is this a job for my PFC (little, sequential and logical) or is this a job for my big guns – giving the non-conscious an opportunity to come up with a solution that is simple, but often brilliant!

Senior leaders at a government agency that I have been working with over the last six months have said to me that even being aware of that choice to park a decision in the midst of daily mayhem has had huge benefits. It greatly reduces their stress associated with decision-making.

Recognise the problems you are solving regularly and ask yourself – do I need to solve this now? Can it wait an hour, a day, a week?

Relax

Insights are connections that are in our brain but, as they're often weak, we don't tend to notice them when we have a busy brain. A crowded brain and insights do not go well together. Therefore, when we are busy, we don't have as many insights as when we have a relaxed brain.

Many of us don't have reflection space in our busy weeks. It's not built-in to our diaries. Most of us have lost all spare spaces in our diaries to meetings, commitments, and emails. We then are connected to the phone and emails even on the way home, and have kids and family commitments until we flake out in the evening (after answering potentially a few more emails)!

But is it possible to rebuild some relaxation time, particularly when you understand that this space is really important? Definitely! It could be in the car on the way to work, or on a bus or on a train; it could be in your exercise regime. A CEO I coached leaves work at 3pm one afternoon a week and goes to the beach, with only a notebook and pen, and that's where he has his greatest insights on steering the company. For me, I've had lots of fantastic brainwaves, ideas, and insights when I am on plane, because it's one of the only places where I'm not connected. Of course, now they have Wi-Fi on the plane, so unless I have the discipline to turn my phone off, I'm going to lose this forced relaxation space. In our busy world, we won't have this time unless we make a commitment to create it.

Without relaxation time, there is little space for innovative ways to build our business or solve our challenges, and we spend all of our time reacting to the day-to-day. It is interesting to test our ability to solve problems and get an understanding of the difference between solving problems logically and solving problems via insight.

As mentioned, Mark Jung-Beeman is an expert in researching insights. The method researchers have used (described above) was known as 'Compound Remote Associate Problems' or... CRAP. For fairly obvious reasons, some people had issues with the acronym, so it's now being called Compound Remote Associates, abbreviated to the rather more G-rated acronym CRA.

I've included some examples below for you to start to practise. You can look them up on Google and do them yourself. For example, see: http://www.remote-associates-test.com. There are puzzles that help promote insights by fostering our ability to make many connections in the brain from remote or disparate things.

- Look at the three words below and come up with one word that goes with each of the three words. Your one word can either go before or after each of the words, and must make a new compound. Just focus on one line at a time[1] (See bottom of the page for the answers)

Cottage	Swiss	Cake
Cream	Skate	Cap
Chocolate	Fortune	Tin
Manners	Round	Tennis
Birthday	Stick	Light

If we have a different cultural or language background, then our connections may be different. Our ability to pull together these words is based on our history of connecting them. For those of us that have a more limited history in our brain, the connections will be fewer.

Similarly, some people's brains make these connections more readily than others. It is to do with openness and the mood we are in, our history, and the way we have stored memories. It's interesting to note, if we practice this exercise in a group and everyone else is getting them, we get ourselves in a bit of a threat state. Our ability to get them is hampered simply by the knowledge that others are getting them while we aren't.

Sometimes we solve them via logic and check the new word against all three words. Sometime it's via insight. When we solve them by insight, our solutions come to us instantly. In our workshops, people put their hand in the air so quickly with a pleased look! Then you can see people thinking "I had better

1 Answers: 1. Cheese 2. Ice 3. Cookie 4. Table 5. Candle. Source: http://www.remote-associates-test.com/

make sure that's right because I didn't check it"; that's how fast our non-conscious brain is working. It had already made enough connections for us to experience a 'knowing' and put our hand up, and we haven't even checked the answer. Our prefrontal cortex (thinking brain) is way behind the action.

Researchers have found that there is a burst of 'alpha waves' at the moment just prior to insights, and a burst of gamma waves at the moment of insight. What does this mean? Before we go onto Reflect, Remove and Reward, let's have a look at brain waves in more detail.

Introducing brain waves

There are five types of brain waves, four of which are important in this context. We have Beta brain waves, which are very fast. They are active when we are talking, thinking and doing in our regular lives. They are measured at approximately 15-30 Hertz. Hertz are used to measure the frequency of electrical impulses across the brain in cycles per second. Alpha brain waves are slower; they are 8-14 Hertz. Then there are Theta brain waves in deep relaxation and Delta brain waves when we are in deep sleep.

Alpha brain waves occur in a quieter brain wave state than the Beta brain waves. When we first wake up in the morning, we shift from more of the Theta/Delta waves to the Alpha waves, and that's when we often have insights. When we are drifting off to sleep, or if we are in a gym or in the shower, we go from busy-busy-busy (Beta) to a quieter brain (Alpha).

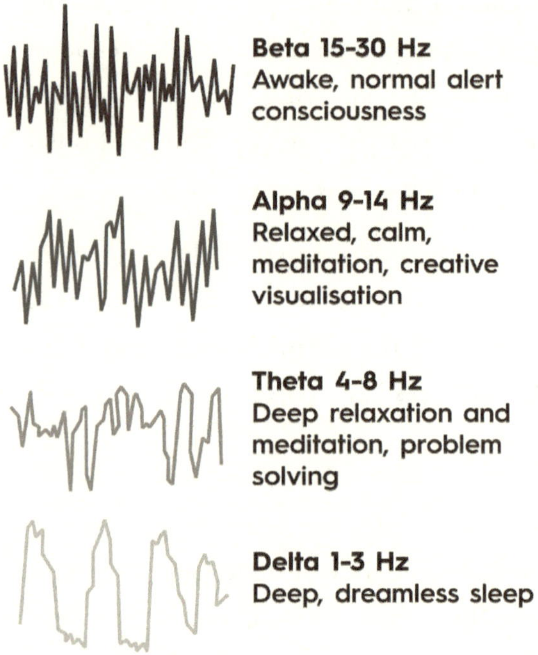

By using an Electroencephalogram [EEG] we can determine which brain waves are present during insight as described above. These distinctive Alpha waves are so related to the state we're in when we get insights that, when a scientist records the Alpha pattern occurring, they can generally predict the person's likelihood of coming up with a novel idea before it actually happens.

Wave	Frequency	Associated Mental State
Gamma	27 Hz and up	Gamma is associated with the formation of ideas, language and memory processing, and various types of learning. Gamma waves have been shown to disappear during deep sleep induced by anaesthesia, but return with the transition back to a wakeful state.

Wave	Frequency	Associated Mental State
Beta	12hz - 27hz	Wide awake. This is the mental state most people are in during the day and most of their waking lives. Usually, this state is uneventful, but don't underestimate its importance. Many people lack sufficient beta activity, which can cause mental or emotional disorders such as depression, ADD and insomnia. And low SMR production (a sub-range of beta at 12-15hz) may be related to insomnia. Stimulating beta activity can improve emotional stability, energy levels, attentiveness and concentration.
Alpha	8hz - 12hz	Awake but relaxed and not processing much information. When you get up in the morning, and just before sleep, you are naturally in this state. When you close your eyes your brain automatically starts producing more alpha waves. Many studies monitoring the EEG activity of experienced meditators have revealed strong increases in alpha activity. Alpha activity has also been connected to the ability to recall memories, have insights, lessened discomfort and pain, and reductions in stress and anxiety.
Theta	3hz - 8hz	Light sleep or extreme relaxation. Theta is also a very receptive mental state that has proven useful for hypnotherapy, as well as self-hypnosis using recorded affirmations and suggestions.

Wave	**Frequency**	**Associated Mental State**
Delta	0.2hz - 3hz	Deep, dreamless sleep. Delta is the slowest band of brainwaves. When your dominant brainwave is delta, your body is healing itself and 'resetting' its internal clocks. You do not dream in this state and are completely unconscious.

18

There are several 'brain entrainment' companies now that sell the benefits of training your brain. You can train to enhance alpha brainwaves to reduce stress and tension, or train to increase beta brainwaves to increase attention and focus. Initial research suggests that this kind of brain exercise does provide benefits, however, as yet, it is unquantified.

Even without formal brain entrainment, we can all increase the amount of alpha brain waves we experience in any given day. If we 'smell the roses', if we close our eyes or if we breathe deeply, we increase alpha brain waves. If we meditate regularly, we can increase alpha brain waves. We can increase a quieter brain state throughout our day by doing these specific things that generate more alpha brain waves, and therefore, more insights. Unfortunately, when we are at work, under pressure, and distracted, we don't focus on such things. We go at a hundred miles an hour, thinking fast with our brain in the beta waves state.

It is only when we consciously look for opportunities to foster the alpha wave brain state that we find them. When we are in a lift, and we are not with somebody else, we can use this transitioning time to breathe deeply, and slow down and quieten the brain-state, rather than racing through our day. Shifting your brain-state makes a huge difference to the amount of insights you have.

Typical triggers that make us feel relaxed are taking a warm shower or bath, exercising, meditation, and driving home. Can you think of any others that work for you? If you have spent all day thinking long and hard about a problem, jumping into the shower can become what scientists call the 'incubation period' for your ideas. Ever followed 'shower thoughts' memes? There's a reason the phrase has stuck! The non-conscious mind has been working extremely hard to solve the problems you face and now that you let your mind wander, it can surface and plant those ideas into your conscious mind.

The chances of having great ideas then are a lot higher. A relaxed state of mind is absolutely crucial to being creative, says Jonah Lehrer, author of *Proust was a Neuroscientist.*

> "Why is a relaxed state of mind so important for creative insights? When our minds are at ease–when those alpha waves are rippling through the brain–we're more likely to direct the spotlight of attention inward, toward that stream of remote associations emanating from the right hemisphere. In contrast, when we are diligently focused, our attention tends to be directed outward, toward the details of the problems we're trying to solve. While this pattern of attention is necessary when solving problems analytically, it actually prevents us from detecting the connections that lead to insights. 'That's why so many insights happen during warm showers,' Bhattacharya says. 'For many people, it's the most relaxing part of the day.' It's not until we're being

massaged by warm water, unable to check our e-mail, that we're finally able to hear the quiet voices in the backs of our heads telling us about the insight. The answers have been there all along–we just weren't listening."[19]

Another key aspect involved in having an insight is distraction, writes Harvard University researcher and psychologist Shelley H. Carson, in her book, Your Creative Brain: '… a distraction may provide the break you need to disengage from a fixation on the ineffective solution.'[20]

Reflect

Helping ourselves and others to increase the Alpha brain-waves

Have you noticed which part of your head you rub when you are stuck thinking "Oh, I can't do this"? We rub our forehead, which is the region of the prefrontal cortex. And why are we rubbing it? Because when we rub it, we get blood flow. We actually know, without knowing it, that rubbing it cause blood-flow. So, if you are stuck in the afternoon, rub your forehead!

What happens when someone comes to you and says, "I have no idea how to solve this problem." You have two options. The easiest and quickest is just to give the person the answer. Many of us are guilty of using this as the main way we deal with team members and their dilemmas. But as discussed earlier, the way to develop the person, to help the other person achieve their own insight and get a surge of dopamine, is to help them solve the problem.

When you ask the person about their thinking, this puts them in a reflection state. Don't ask what they are going to do about it, but rather, what are they thinking about it?

But what if they give an answer like: "I don't know. I haven't thought about it at all. I just came straight to you with the problem."

That's another opportunity. You could say:

- "Well, let's do some thinking."
- "What sort of thinking is important for you to consider regarding this problem?"
- "What thinking have you been doing about this?"
- "How have you been thinking about this?"
- "When you think about this situation, what is coming to mind?"

What we want to do is to get people into their reflective state, increase their alpha brain waves, and encourage them to have an insight and come up with the answer themselves.

Remember: if a person gets an insight, at that point she is motivated to act because dopamine encourages it. Dopamine not only makes her feel good; it also gives her a propensity to move. Dopamine is a motivating neurochemical.

So far we've understood that we need to be in a quiet, reflective state. But what on earth do I mean by suggesting we shouldn't focus directly on the problem?

Remove

Here's an example; I ask a staff member, Sarah, to tell me what is causing her concern after a flat "all right" in response to my question, "How's things?" Then I proceed to ask her about the problem, which she explains is related to a colleague not completing their tasks on time. If I go on to ask Sarah all about the detail of that problem, such as "What tasks?" and "When were they supposed to be completed?", I am showing empathy to Sarah, but we are also both still focussed heavily on the problem.

Where else could I focus if not on the problem? There are two possibilities: focus on Sarah's thinking, and focus on the solution. What is it that Sarah really wants from her colleagues and the project task and timing? What is her thinking?

Instead of doing what many managers do – which is to ask a lot of questions about the problem out of a desire to solve the problem – we might be more vigilant. We step into that leadership space, and we say instead, "Sarah, what outcome are you after?" "What thinking have you done around how to improve the situation?" "How might you communicate that with your colleague?" We are then supporting Sarah to solve her own problem.

This is the crucial moment. It's at this point that many managers come in with their own ideas. But this is when we want people to come up with their own good ideas and to think outside the square about what else could they do.

What do I focus on? I spend more time on the solution and her thinking than the actual description of the problem. This way,

Sarah has more chances to move into the reward state; she is already imagining a great outcome for the project. If we think about it, when people come to describe a problem to us, they are already in a slight threat state. If we focus more and more on the problem, they stay in a threat state. And if they are in the threat state, they won't have a chance to get an insight.

Alice Flaherty, renowned neuroscientist and author of The Midnight Disease (a book about the neural basis of creativity), show us that this approach creates a virtuous cycle. Reaching our own insights gives us a surge of dopamine, and dopamine is a very important ingredient in our creativity. The more dopamine that is released, the more creative we are. Flaherty writes: "People vary in terms of their level of creative drive according to the activity of the dopamine pathways of the limbic system."

Reward

Moving out of threat state into reward

We've acknowledged that when we are faced with a dilemma we are often in a threat state. Knowing that this is unlikely to produce an insight can motivate us to shift this state quickly, at least to neutral, if not to a reward state. We are going to cover a quick 30 second circuit breaker in the next section in REGULATE, which will help you shift from threat to reward.

You can help the person get to a reward state just by the tone of your questions. Here are some samples of the type of questions or statements that will get them there:

- "You know you've come to this sort of problem before. What were your thoughts previously?"
- "I think you are really talented at this."
- "You know your customers really well."
- "You know the situation really well."

Asking these questions or making these suggestions is more likely to put someone in a reward state.

One other key way to do this is to focus on the outcome or goal we are after. We often get bogged down in the detail and drama of a problem and catastrophise it, but if we can turn our attention back toward our purpose, mission, goal or outcome, we can quite easily experience more of a reward state as we imagine that future position.

A colleague of mine is using this concept to shift the focus in Healthcare away from "Stopping bullying!" to "Create positive work environments!" Dr Cath Crock, a physician and expert on culture change in healthcare, has seen first-hand the drastic change you can bring about with a solution-focused approach. "Instead of focussing on bullying, harassment, or bad behaviour in healthcare, a more positive approach is to look to the future we would all prefer - a kind health system - one that is kind to those working in it and kind to those receiving the care."

Dr Crock tells a story of a child with chronic illness who was in the hospital frequently for operations. The child's father had been labelled by staff members as aggressive, and security had been called on him a number of times for causing disturbances in the operating room. Dr Crock spoke to the father before his son's next operation, and asked "Can I do anything for you? What do you need to feel relaxed while your son is in theatre?" The father broke down and said that he was very upset every time his son had an operation, because he wasn't able to pray for him. Dr Crock showed the father where the hospital chapel was, and the staff waited for his return to begin the operation. Since then, this family has been heartfelt in their support of the hospital, and the staff enjoy working with them. The relationship has improved for all involved simply by focussing on the solution that was needed – a way for the father to feel relaxed during a stressful procedure.

CHAPTER FIVE

Multi-tasking

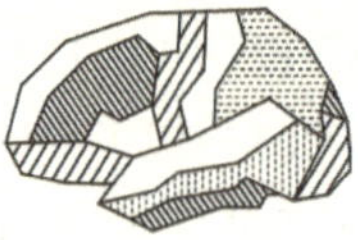

In business today, many people multi-task, and many people are proud of it. Multi-tasking has been on the rapid rise with our always-on technology, the need to do more with less time and resources, and the belief that it is more productive. This could mean typing an email while still talking on the phone, answering emails in the middle of writing a proposal, talking with somebody while reading a text message, or writing notes on an unrelated topic while talking on the phone. It seems most people embark on some form of multi-tasking in the vain attempt to get through everything in their day. In particular, people struggle with their emails, so the idea that a few quick emails could be attended to while talking on the phone to a colleague, client, or direct report is appealing.

Multitasking, in the neuroscience world, is actually called 'switching'. Even this linguistic difference gives us a clue – are we actually doing multiple things at once, or just moving between multiple things? Switching is very fast information flow from the right hemisphere to the left hemisphere through the corpus callosum. The corpus callosum is the only part of our brain that joins the left and right hemispheres. Imagine them as two separate, distinct halves, with the corpus callosum joining them. Information can only flow as fast as this thin pathway allows.

Research also shows that multitasking lowers your IQ. A study at the University of London found that participants who multitasked during cognitive tasks experienced IQ score declines that were similar to what they'd expect if they had smoked marijuana and stayed up all night. Men experienced IQ drops of 15 points while multitasking, lowering their scores to the average range of an 8-year-old child![21] I like to cheekily suggest in workshops that men are better off smoking marijuana and staying up all night. If they did that, and didn't multi-task instead, no-one would tell the difference!

For women, they only lose five IQ points when they multi-task, because their corpus callosum has been described by one of my lecturers as a multi-lane highway. Men's corpus callosum, by comparison, is a "little English country laneway".

This also is explained when you look at the difference between the connectomes (neural pathways) in men's, and women's, brains. A man's brain connects, more often, front to back and a women's brain from side to side.

But that doesn't mean that multitasking is a good idea for anyone. It usually takes 25% longer to complete the tasks when we multitask, and it increases our stress level when we multitask. These are two findings that clearly show us that multitasking is

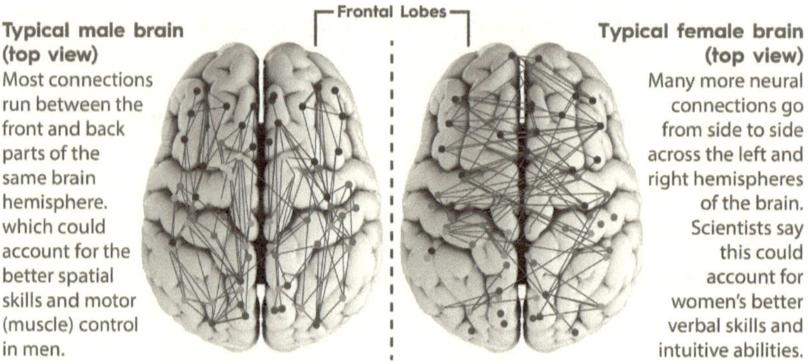

http://www.independent.co.uk, 2013

not ideal. We think it improves our productivity, but it actually doesn't, it reduces it.

As multi-tasking drains a lot of mental and physical energy, we feel like we're productive – we worked hard and used energy so we must have produced a lot. However, just because we expend energy does not mean we are productive – it only creates an illusion of productivity.

A study at the Institute of Psychiatry by Hewlett Packard found excessive use of technology reduced workers' intelligence. They found those distracted by incoming email and phone calls saw a 10-point fall in their IQ – more than twice that found in studies of the impact of smoking marijuana. However, this drop was not a permanent drop and related more to the ongoing distraction of email.[22]

Let's say we are writing a programme, a proposal or a strategic document. If we then also get emails popping in all the time and we check them in the middle of our writing, it will slow us down significantly. It turns us from one way of thinking into another, and switching between different tasks is very draining for the brain.

> Funny, I just realised I have had three pop-up messages from my open Skype with a colleague about catching up with her when I am next in Brisbane. I've now turned Skype off to finish my editing on this book!

Multi-tasking doesn't allow for 'deep work'

Georgetown Professor Cal Newport thinks uninterrupted, distraction-free deep work is so important that if you're unable to do this at your current job, you should start looking for another.

Newport suggests this is where 'deep work' comes in, which is "when you focus without distraction on a cognitively demanding task. For an effort to be considered deep work—and for it to reap the rewards depth can offer—there can be no distraction." That means not even a quick glance at your inbox, which can "drastically reduce your cognitive function and therefore reduce the quality and quantity of what you produce."[23]

> Research shows it takes an average of 64 seconds to recover train of thought after checking email
>
> Check every 5 mins = waste 8.5 per hours per week
>
> **(Jackson, Dawson @ Wilson)**

The brain prefers to work on one type of task for a period of time. If you are working on strategy, work on strategy. If you are then answering twenty emails, answer twenty emails. If you are then doing something creative, do something creative. Try to lock in things for the diary schedule, rather than getting halfway through a strategic discussion with somebody, and then doing something creative. Our brains prefer to do one thing.

When we are multi-tasking we are actually attention switching. It only appears we are doing multiple things simultaneously. However, in this switching we experience an "attentional blink". We lose time, a lag time of 200 to 500 milliseconds (0.5 second) between activities. In this time, we miss information such as body language cues and subtle emotional changes. We are not mindful and not present.

This process also increases our stress significantly as we move from one thing to the next in quick succession. The more we inhibit throughout the day, the less we have the ability to inhibit. This is another explanation of why our pre-frontal cortex seems to run out of gas later in the day.

Why we like getting distracted

Curiosity

Why does our brain want to get distracted by emails? We get drawn to the emails by our curiosity. Neurochemicals - dopamine and norepinephrine - are released when we discover something new and we don't know what it is. We are drawn to find out.

That email could mean we have won a million dollars! Or it might mean someone is taking the burden that we have had for months off our back. Nine times out of ten they are giving us a burden, but on the off-chance that there is going to be some great news, we take a look at the email.

Status

Another reason we check our email is because we are highly relational people; we love that someone wants us. If we are getting an email, we are also getting a dopamine hit because we feel we are important; there is somebody who needs us for something and that feels good.

Habit

The more you answer the emails as they come, the more you are wiring yourself to habitually answer emails. Then, even if you don't think about it, even if you aren't excited about a new email, even if you are really proactively wanting to stay focused on writing the proposal, your finger has already gone to that email. You have trained yourself that whenever there is a 'ding' it means check your emails.

What to do instead

People who use their brain more effectively are better at inhibiting those tendencies and saying to themselves, "I will come back to that later; now is not the time to do this, I have a task I am already working on."

Alternatively, we can retrain ourselves so that 'ding', means park that email and come back to it. Or even better than that, we tweak our environment to stop those triggers. I don't have the ding on my laptop. My phone doesn't even vibrate when I get an email or text message. I have to actively look at it every now and then if I want to see a message. Because I have the tendency to look and I don't have the skills to inhibit myself, why should I put myself under that pressure?

Inhibiting also takes energy

Unfortunately, every time we inhibit, we use up a little bit of that resource that we could use for something more important, something clever. Another good technique is to turn off the monitor on our screen when we are doing something that requires us to stay on task, so we won't see that little star on the envelope in the corner of the screen. Some companies are only pushing or pulling email through certain hours. Some organisations have moved from 10am-12noon and 2pm-4pm for emails to get pushed-through. If you send email outside those hours, you get a message that says, "I do not receive/see my email outside these hours, if you need an answer outside these hours, please phone." These companies are trying to limit that continuous email bombardment, because they understand that this switching is not productive.

CHAPTER SIX

Peak Mental Performance

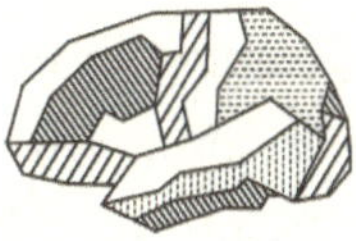

With the amount of pressure we are under to answer emails and attend meetings, we are left with very little time to create, strategise, innovate, think, develop and plan. For many of us our day starts and ends with emails, we email continuously, we attend back-to-back meetings and we multi-task in the vain attempt to complete everything we need to in the day. Overall we are still left feeling overwhelmed and out of control.

To achieve peak performance, we need to re-engineer our day. We need to bring back prioritising as the first thing we do each day. We need some reflection time and brain breaks, and we need to do one thing at a time, preferably in a reward state. 'Chunking' time refers to doing like things together. If we are writing, write articles and reports. If we doing administration, then file and answer simple emails. If we are working on a strategy document and need to be strategic, set aside this time as strategic time. We tend, instead, to be writing a strategy document while we are regularly interrupted with random emails of various topics and then we answer some calls in the middle of it all. This is not giving us optimal brain function. We are multi-tasking and not staying in single mode at one time.

The illustration below is the summary of the Effective and Ineffective habits of our daily leadership lives. Most people that I have been training identify not just with one or two bad habits, but with all of them.

Some companies have now moved to 20 and 45 minute meetings to replace 30 and 60 minute meetings in an attempt to be more efficient in meetings. It also allows team members time to mentally and physically prepare for the next meeting and perhaps even have a brain-break between meetings. One senior executive, after implementing this for a month with his whole team, said now he's thrilled to look into his diary and see the many 15 minutes in which he can go to the bathroom! This is a feat in today's crazy corporate and organisational world.

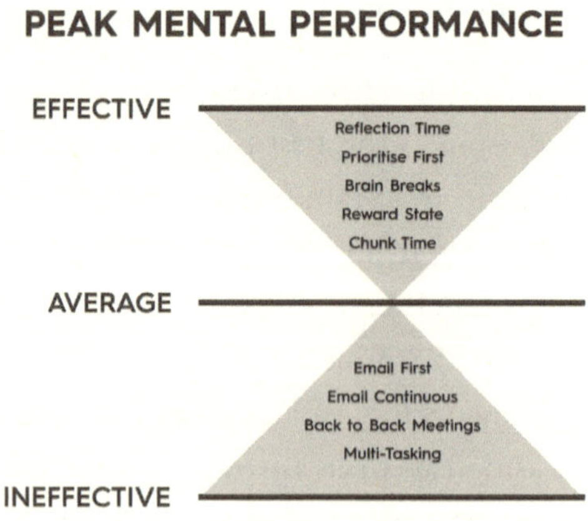

Source: Enhansen Performance

Brain-breaks

According to Tony Schwartz, CEO of The Energy Project, most people hold their productivity back by not rigidly scheduling work & rest breaks throughout the day.[24]

We need to have brain breaks every 1.5 hours. If we take a break regularly we recharge our PFC, which has a cumulative effect during the day regarding our capacity later in the day.

Prioritising

One of the best habits to get into relates to email. Refrain from opening your email before you have thought about what you want to get done each day. We might not remember everything and our inbox may change what we need to do, but actually thinking, proactively and intentionally, about the three or four most important things to do today can transform our productivity.

Then, after we've planned how to make time for these important things, we go into emails and do the truly urgent ones. We can do what needs to be done with email in 30-45 minutes. It's a real discipline and not easy to do, but people who move towards having a good discipline over their day, rather than letting their inbox rule their entire existence, get a lot more done. They also feel less stressed. Our email can make us feel out of control, as if we don't have a say in what we do all day. Even the process of thinking and prioritising the three things we need to complete each day makes us feel more focused. The trap is not to choose too many priorities, because your day may already be full.

I worked with a client who was an international manager for a large global travel company. When I met her for the first time, she said "My entire life is controlled by emails." She was concerned, as was her manager, that she was not prioritising the strategic part of her large role. She needed to take charge and be the one deciding when and how long to email for, rather than just continuously being on email from the minute she woke up till late into the night. She needed to delegate and spend less time on each email. She also needed to let some people know that her response time would be longer than she would have normally responded in. She was stressed and anxious when I met her. It was taking a toll on her well-being.

After we had put in new, brain-based strategies she became more disciplined about prioritising first thing in the day. As part of that prioritising, she worked out what she could delegate. She then built in time in her diary to the important things, turned off her email for 30 minutes while completing important tasks, and gave herself time limits around email correspondence. She found she could gain a sense of control and she was able to work on strategy. She was no longer stressed and stretched despite still having a massive workload, and her manager was very positive with the results.

When leaders give their permission for teams not to be ruled by emails they create a productive culture. When we, as leaders, says let's prioritise time for ourselves, for reflection, and for creative strategy, it is much more effective. We let our staff know that if they haven't heard from somebody for a while, they can pick up the phone. Give permission for your teams to not be ruled by email.

Reflecting

Reflection time may involve booking a meeting room for half an hour and going there with our pen and paper. Some people put reflection time in to their diary and don't allow anything else to be booked, giving them some space to think. One of the senior managers that I work with decided to do some reflection time as he drives to work. He turns off the radio and all distractions. He is proactive about using this time to think and plan for the next three to six months. We can all find our own way to build in reflection time.

Chunking

Chunking is the process of breaking up your day into larger chunks instead of continuously doing many small things while reacting to constant interruptions. The more you chunk your time, the more you can devote undivided attention to specific tasks. It will also mean you have shorter start-up times and your efficiency improves significantly. Since you won't be spending as much time in start-up moments, you will get more done. As you will be able to focus on the single task at hand, you will do it better, faster and experience less stress. You will also feel like you are accomplishing more as you are setting smaller goals and achieving them.

Start by chunking just 20 or 30 minutes to complete a particular task or project. Later you can chunk your day in up to 90 minute sections at times where that is appropriate. Let people around you know that you need some un-interrupted time to complete something.

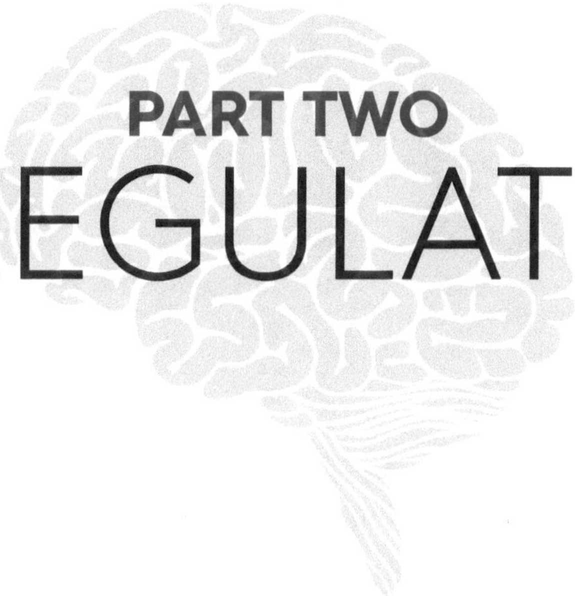

PART TWO
REGULATE

CHAPTER SEVEN

Arousal stress and peak performance

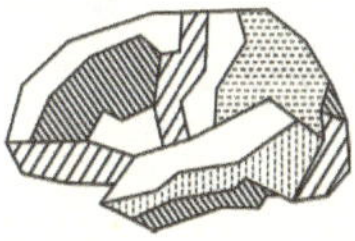

Once we understand how we Think and how our brain chemistry responds to stimulus, we are in a position to Regulate our emotions. Of course, understanding how we think is the biggest part of applying the TREAD framework, because we cover all of the key elements of brain. We can use that knowledge about the brain to regulate responses and reactions. We have all the principles that are going to feed all the other elements of TREAD – Regulate, Engage, Adapt and Develop.

It's important to remember that some degree of 'arousal stress' is required for us to get to peak performance. When I am talking about arousal stress, I mean neurochemical transmission. According to Dr Evian Gordon, CEO and Chairman of MyBrainSolution.com, 'Stress is the activation of your 'fight-flight reflex' when your body perceives itself to be in a threatening situation. Chronic stress narrows your focus of attention, damages your brain and reduces your immune functions." Everybody is

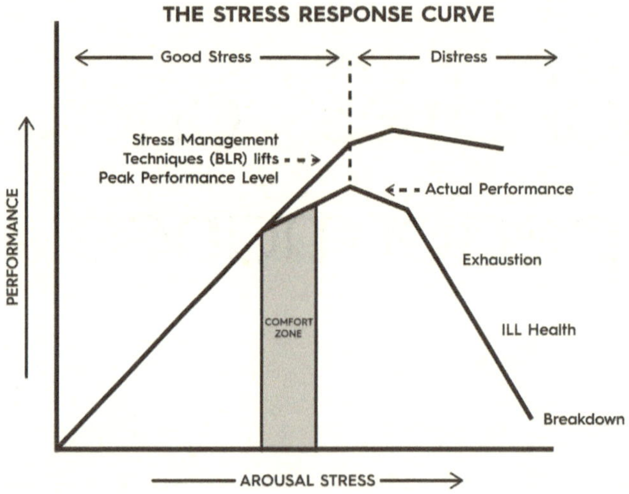

Source: Enhansen Performance

different when it comes to the right amount of arousal stress. Some people achieve peak performance with less arousal stress, so their curves on this diagram would be flatter. Some people's curves are taller. The point I am making is that we're in our comfort zone just before we reach our peak performance. What we need is a bit of a stretch, a bit of a tweak, to get to our peak performance.

It is useful to look at some of the key differences that have been identified when it comes to men, women, and their brains.

Amy Arnsten found that men, on average, sit in the comfort zone regarding performance naturally. They are almost at the top near peak performance, but need more arousal stress to get to peak performance. She also found that women, on average, sit more typically on the top of the arousal curve, meaning they are more likely to go over the edge and move into distress than their male counterparts. However, each man and women is very different and we could never generalise based on this.There are many men and women who sit elsewhere on the curve (needing more or less arousal stress for peak performance).

Usually when I get people to guess the point where men and women sit on average, a majority of people get it right for men (just below peak performance) and most suggest that women on average are over the peak and already at over-arousal.

There are a number of other specific anatomical and functional differences between the sexes listed in the table below.

Anatomical and functional differences exist between the brains of men and women: [25]

	Women's Brain	**Men's Brain**
Anatomical	- More interconnected than male brains. - Larger hippocampal size (pertaining to better spatial relationship and navigation). - Frontal Cortex (cognitive functions) is more flexible in women than men. - Limbic Cortex (emotional processing) is larger and more active in females than males.	- More lateralized than female brains. - Men Parietal Cortex (more active in spatial processing). - Greater right amygdala function contributing to greater arousal (especially to novel stimuli).

	Women's Brain	Men's Brain
Functional	- Increased left amygdala activity corresponds to a greater ability with greater emotional recognition. - Lower threshold of vigilance of signals indicating danger. - Enhanced Verbal Memory.	- Increased ability to recognise anger.

Men often sit to the left of the peak, which means we can put a little bit more pressure on them to get them into peak performance and out of their comfort zone. For men, we can help them to achieve their peak performance by saying: "I think you can jump a little bit higher, and even a bit higher than that."

Men deal with that pressure, on average, a little bit better than women do. Why is that? Women often sit right at the peak of the performance curve! Which looks great, but there is a problem with that. Women can go over the edge. Women don't always perform as well when we apply more pressure.

Of course, this is an average bell curve. We will find that some men respond to pressure and some don't; some women will achieve their peak under more pressure, and some won't. We cannot just assume that we need to stretch men and pussyfoot around the women, because it's not true. As leaders, we need to know where each of our team members sits on the performance curve as an individual. It's useful to understand that there can be a difference between gender.

Think about where you sit on the peak performance curve. Ask yourself, do I need more arousal stress to perform at my best? Or do I perform at my peak when I am less stressed?

Stressed, but not too stressed

The interesting concept to understand about the peak performance curve is to be clear about when the prefrontal cortex gets to its maximum capability. We want to apply just the right amount of arousal stress to ourselves and our teams, but not too much. We know what happens when we are too stressed. We flip into the threat state, and we start to underperform.

Once we discover our limits, it's tempting to stay in our comfort zone and not to get too stressed. But if we never push our limits, then we don't reach our potential. The best solution is to learn to push ourselves, recognise when we have gone too far, and recover. When our amygdala is over aroused, we want to get out of that state straight away. How can we do that? By learning a 30-second 'circuit breaker'.

CHAPTER EIGHT

The 30-second circuit breaker

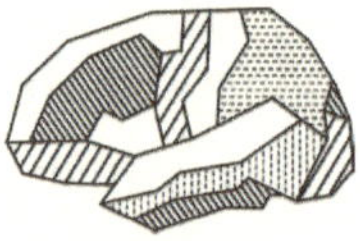

This is a simple strategy to apply when we get into a threat state. It is called 'Breathe – Label – Reappraise', or BLR for short, because we need something simple for the brain to remember when we sense a threat. In fact, most of my clients shorten it even further by calling it "bla" – "I just Bla" – which is great as a very quick reference.

Breathe

Here is a personal example. Some mornings when I drive in to work or to the airport, I feel a sense of threat. I don't know why, but I think it has to do with Sydney traffic. You just never know if there is going to be a truck stuck in the tunnel because they were too high. This has happened a number of times and it creates chaos for hours. There is no way of making it to the airport on time when this has happened. What I do know is that I need to BLR. I start by inhaling and exhaling slowly.

This simple step makes a huge difference to our sense of threat for two reasons. Deep breathing:

1. Pumps oxygen to the prefrontal cortex. That oxygen helps us inhibit and regulate our fight-flight-freeze response.

2. Slows down our heart rate. The more we do deep breathing, the more we increase our heart rate variability – our ability to regulate our heart rate. If we increase our heart rate variability, we increase our overall immune system strength. Heart rate variability increases resilience.

Essentially, every time we breathe deeply, we activate our parasympathetic nervous system – the part of our nervous system that is calming.

Think of a car on a hill. We have an activation part of our body, the accelerator, known as our sympathetic nervous system. Our parasympathetic nerve system is our clutch. If we keep the clutch part way out, we are not going anywhere. We might be over-revving, but we are not going anywhere. That's a big waste of our energy. We start wasting all our fuel and then, when we do want to take off at peak performance, we can't. What peak performance leaders do is look at how we activate when we need to, and how to come off – using the clutch effectively – when we need to.

The aim of our central nervous system is to help our body stay in homeostasis – which is remaining stable and constant – so that when we activate it, we can also pull ourselves back. That's the balance between on and off.

Think about elite athletes. They don't train for days and hours on end without a break. Their schedule allows for breaks in between, even if they are training intensely. They go hard and then they pull back. They go hard and they pull back. To become a 'corporate athlete' and achieve peak performance is a matter of learning to go hard, but also to pull back.

My Calm Beat is an app that you can get on your phone. It's free, and it helps us breathe at the right breathing rate: six breaths per minute. This is a breath rate that really triggers your parasympathetic nervous system to slow down. Everybody has a 'best breathing rate' somewhere between 4.5 and seven breaths per minute. Once My Calm Beat comes on, it helps you breathe at six breaths per minute (a suggested median breathing rate by Dr Evian Gordon if you don't know your personal best breathing rate). This trains us to do deep breathing.

Just 10 minutes of slow, deep breathing like that, even in chunks of two minutes, lasts you — resilience wise — for 24 hours.

Dr Evian Gordon says, 'You will not only be more calm on the day you train, but you will lower the threshold at which you activate your fight-flight reflex. With training, you also increase your 'flexible decision making and adaptive vagus system.' As calmness training becomes an automatic daily habit, you will increasingly deepen this brain network, and be more calm and in the moment before any stressful situation.'

A neuroscientist that I work with suggests that we breathe out first, not in. The reason for that is that when we are stressed or angry, it takes prefrontal cortex involvement to breathe out. We automatically breathe in, but breathing out engages the prefrontal cortex.

Label

After we breathe, we then label the emotion. Labelling the emotion means giving it a name, an emotional tag. We use our prefrontal cortex to give our feelings a name. When we are feeling angry, annoyed, frustrated, we label it. For example:

> Exhale: 'Okay, I'm feeling a bit overwhelmed now.'
>
> Inhale: 'Breathing deeply.'

What's the benefit of labelling? Why is it so useful? It serves two purposes for us. One, it simply switches on our prefrontal cortex, engaging our rational thoughts rather than just relying on emotions. Two, it allows us to externalise. We can step back from the feelings we're having, and view and assess them more objectively. It takes us from being at the mercy of our feelings to being far more in control. We can't make choices about what to do with our feelings until we recognise what they are. Curiously, even the act of naming a feeling, of establishing what it is that's making you feel bad, can be enough to make you feel much better.

Reappraise

Once our breath has helped to calm us down, and we gain some insight into our feelings by labelling them, it's time to ask ourselves a question: "How else can I look at this?" More specifically, we can ask:

> 'Can I see the positive in this?'
>
> 'What can I learn from this?'
>
> 'What will I gain from this?'
>
> 'What can I be thankful for?'
>
> 'How big an issue is this in the scheme of things?'
>
> 'In five years, is this 10 minutes going to matter?'

Any of those questions help us reappraise. I love that whenever we really need to, we can always pull in a 'big' reappraisal. Victor Frankel was a prisoner in the concentration camps in Nazi Germany in the Second World War. He wrote a book called In Man's Search For Meaning which, by his death in 1997, had sold over 10 million copies and was translated into 24 languages.

Frankel's book is all about reappraisal. Although he lost many close family members, his physical freedom, clothes, and house, Frankel concludes that a prisoner's psychological reactions are not only the result of the conditions but the freedom of choice he always has mentally, even in terrible conditions. This is based on having a hope for the future, about reappraising and focussing on that possible future, and living in the moment.

Frankel really harnessed the power of reappraisal in the extreme circumstances that he found himself in. Fortunately, we don't have to reappraise that hard every day. But we all face difficult events from time to time, when we need to bring in the big guns. We might even say, "Thank goodness I've got a healthy family; thank goodness I live in Australia." Sometimes we need throw in ideas like that to reappraise.

Breathe – Label – Reappraise (BLR) is a simple 30-second fix to use when we realise we are being controlled by our emotions. Calm that amygdala down by breathing, labelling, and talking to yourself for 30 seconds about re-thinking what's going on in your head.

In order to build our resilience, we don't just need a "bounce back" strategy such as BLR when we experience negative emotions. We also need to ensure we are doing things in our life that support our ability to bounce back. Mindfulness practise, brain-breaks, the right diet, sleep and exercise are all elements that contribute to building our resilience. We will look into these further.

CHAPTER NINE

Mindfulness

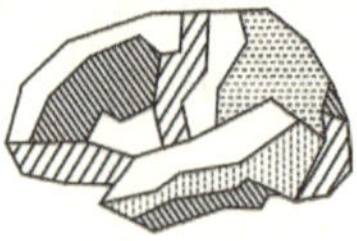

Using the BLR strategy takes awareness – or mindfulness. We need to know when to use BLR, and it takes mindfulness to say, "How am I feeling right now? Do I need to calm myself down, make myself feel at ease, get myself in the reward state?"

If we are never mindful of how we are feeling, we won't think to use the BLR strategy. If we can learn to be more aware of the emotions we are experiencing, then we can use BLR every time we experience a slight threat state. In that 30 seconds, our limbic system goes down and our cognitive ability goes up again. A lot of managers I have worked with use BLR regularly.

A CEO recently contacted me and said, "You saved my life with BLR. We had to close the entire factory, 140 people, and I personally did a lot of the communication with those people who had been retrenched. I BLR'd and BLR'd and BLR'd all day long, and it really helped me."

Let's look a little more deeply at mindfulness. This practice is proven to be fantastic for the brain. Mindfulness exercises actually increase the brain matter in the prefrontal cortex. In particular, it increases our ability to regulate emotions. So, mindfulness practice is now understood as a powerful tool in regulating our stress emotions.

There is a bit of a misconception around mindfulness, about it being soft and fluffy and head in the clouds. Mindfulness is not about going off to LaLaLand. Mindfulness is about being present. The definition of mindfulness is paying attention to now.

That's not easy to do. It takes practice. Our brains are always thinking about the past, and thinking about the future. If you quiet your brain right now, you'll notice that you start thinking about your emails or what you said to someone this morning, what you are going to have for lunch or that you forgot to take the meat out of the freezer for dinner. Your brain will automatically return to the 'default network' – which is also called the narrative circuitry. Our brains tell a little story, and it goes on and on.

Direct experience – being present – is when you smell the roses. Direct experience is when you use any of your senses in the present. When we are listening to our breath and feeling it through our nostrils, we are in direct experience. Mindfulness is paying attention to your senses as a way of being present. Default is what we do automatically. If we want to calm our brain down and build our resilience, then we do a bit of mindfulness practice.

There is a lot of help available to develop this practice. A great app called Headspace takes you through a 10-minute guided mindfulness exercise every day. You don't need to do a mindfulness exercise for long amounts of time for it to benefit you. You just need to practice it consistently.

To help me remember how to practice mindfulness, I use the ABCD of Mindfulness model. This model is created by the founders of the PotentialProject.com.

> A is for anatomy. Sit comfortably in a neutral position.
>
> B is for breathing. The type of breathing is a relaxed deep breath.
>
> C is for counting. Count to 10, one on every out breath, and when you get to ten, count back to 1. Do 10 breaths up and 10 back down.
>
> D is for distraction. We always have distractions. "What's for lunch? Oh, this is interesting, I hadn't thought of that, I need to do this and that." That is normal. Notice the distraction, and bring yourself back to the present.

The practice of mindfulness involves repeatedly bringing ourselves back to our breath and our counting. Focus your attention on your breath, the feeling of it in your nose, the sound of it, and the sound of your counting: one, two ...

This is a simple mindfulness practice. If you have never done mindfulness, the counting helps because otherwise we drift off into our default thinking for five minutes before we say whoops and come back to the breath. That doesn't work. We become frustrated and we give up because we think we can't 'do mindfulness'. But if we pay attention to counting, we notice as soon as we become distracted as we can hear the counting in the background. Mindfulness is not about 'not getting distracted'. Mindfulness is about being able to recognise your distraction, and put it out of your mind. You don't do it once, and then think "I've succeeded!" It's a process you do over and over again, developing your strength of mindfulness as a skill.

This is a just an introduction to mindfulness. There are a great many wonderful resources, online and in books, to help you develop a mindfulness practice. Many managers have used the apps Headspace or Smiling Minds with great success.

CHAPTER TEN

Diet, sleep and exercise

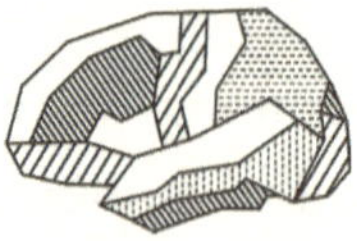

The trifecta of peak performance

Diet, sleep and exercise all impact our peak performance.

The research behind all of these is absolutely fascinating. Here are just a few examples.

1. A 10-minute nap will deliver three hours of reinvigorated prefrontal cortex capability.

2. In yoga, when we are in a position that is awkward for our body and we try to hold it and breathe, we are actually training our brain to get out of a threat state. It's training us to be calm under pressure. It's amazing to think that's what yoga is doing! It is a mental-over-physical scenario. We can use breathing to find that sense of calm, and transition out of that threat state.

3. Carbohydrates – which we find in foods like bread and pasta – can make us tired because they trigger a surge of the brain chemical, serotonin. If you get sleepy after a big meal of carbohydrates, be mindful if you have a task in the afternoon where you need to be alert.

The sleeping brain

How much sleep is the right amount of sleep? What the science finds is that we are all different. There is a bell curve. Most of us would sleep between seven and nine hours a night. Some range between five and 10 hours.

You might think you can function well on just a few hours' sleep, but if you need to sleep in a lot on the weekend, then you are not getting enough sleep during weeknights. However, if you wake every day refreshed from five hours of sleep that may be all you need. The ideal amount of sleep is when you wake up automatically, no alarm. What time do you need to go to bed in order to wake up without your alarm? Now that's an interesting thought!

Although sleep appears to be a passive and restful time, it actually involves a highly active and well-scripted interplay of brain circuits, resulting in sleep's various stages. These stages were discovered in the 1950s through experiments using electroencephalography (EEG) to examine human brain waves. During sleep, the cerebral cortex is rippled by slow waves, i.e., between 0.5 and 4.5 Hz, and this is helpful to recharge our brain.

Professor Leon Lack, sleep scientist at Flinders University in Adelaide says, "A brief nap can not only reduce sleepiness, but also improve cognitive functioning and psychomotor performance (the brain telling the body to move). A few minutes of shut-eye also considerably enhances short-term memory and mood."[26]

Seven-minute workout apps

The science shows that seven minutes of high cardio activity can be really effective for the brain and for the body. The secret is to exercise hard, and I have to warn you: this kind of exercise often includes 'burpees' (jumping into a push-up from a squat and leaping into the air afterwards!)

The 'Scientific 7-Minute Workout', devised by fitness writer Gretchen Reynolds, includes 12 different exercises: jumping jacks, wall sits, push-ups, abdominal crunches, chair step-ups, squats, triceps dips on chair, planks, high knees running in place, lunges, push-up and rotations, and side planks. The interesting part of this exercise plan is it doesn't need any machine or exercise tools. Your only required equipment is a chair and a wall!

Donovan Green, celebrity fitness trainer and author of No Excuses Fitness told Medical Daily:

> "They can do it at home or at work. Seven minutes is easier to do and is more efficient than a one-hour workout. It will boost your metabolism and increase strength during the workout. To see similar fitness and cardiovascular benefits, you can do calisthenics to martial arts."[27]

Even two-and-a-half minutes of high-intensity exercise can be as effective as running for 90 minutes at a moderate pace, according to a study conducted by researchers from Aberdeen University. The research team explained that high-intensity interval training encourages the liver to absorb more fat from blood before using it. Work by scientists at McMaster University in Hamilton, Ontario, shows that even a few minutes of training at an intensity approaching your maximum capacity produces molecular changes within muscles comparable to those of several hours of running or bike riding.[28]

It is well-established that exercise increases perfusion (pushing blood into our capillaries). Since the brain depends on oxygen and glucose, anything that enhances their delivery to brain tissue will consequently facilitate neuroplasticity.[29] Neuroplasticity also improves with the development of synaptic connections and neural networks. These structural and functional changes enhance learning and, ultimately, create a more efficient brain with a greater capacity to learn.[30] When we bring together diet, sleep, and exercise, we have more balance, and we build resilience.

Brain breaks

Schwartz cites a research study conducted by the Federal Aviation Administration that revealed how short breaks between longer working sessions resulted in a 16% improvement in awareness & focus.

> "Research from Peretz Lavie on ultradian rhythms matches up with these findings: longer productive sessions (of 90

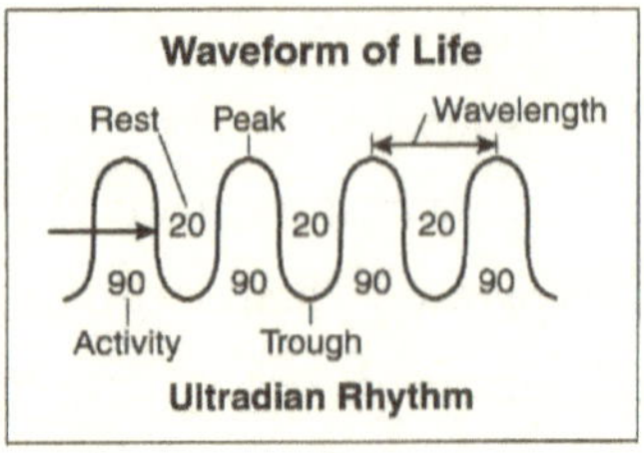

minutes) followed by short breaks (of no more than 15-20 minutes) sync more closely with our natural energy cycles and allow us to maintain a better focus and higher energy level throughout the day".[31]

Ensuring we have a strategy to bounce back from negative emotions as well providing ourselves with a holistic approach to well-being, gives us the best chance of regulating emotions, managing stress and being more resilient. It's useful to regularly ask ourselves what we could be doing to improve these various aspects.[32]

PART THREE
Engage

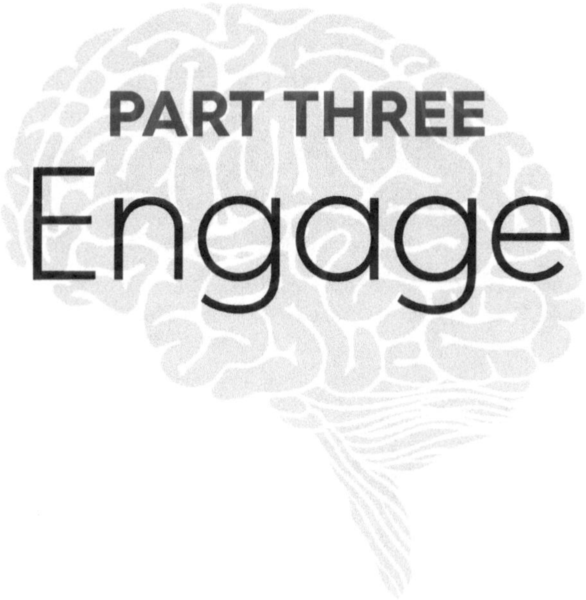

CHAPTER ELEVEN

Engagement in the workplace

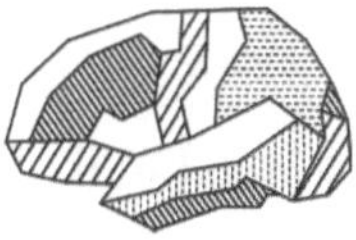

So far, we have looked at how we think, and how we regulate ourselves – our self-leadership. We are now ready to look at engagement, relationships and performance in relation to leading others.

In ENGAGE, we look at what it takes to engage our team members. We start by understanding engagement and its measures, before moving onto emotion contagion. Next we'll look at the social motivators that most impact whether team members will be in a threat or a reward state during or after an interaction.

In our workshops, we then take the concept of engagement to include high performing teamwork, and facilitate around the following questions:

What are high performing teams? Is your team high performing?

What do they need to do to be high performing?

What can leaders of teams do to engage their team members to operate at a high performing level?

How do leaders continuously evolve their teams so they are improving and being agile in the face of disruption and change?

How do you motivate teams during this time?

Understanding engagement

Of massive interest over recent years has been this notion of engagement. Many people are not engaged in their work, coming in simply to clock on and clock off, and are therefore not emotionally committed to improving their performance.

Nowadays, companies are regularly measuring their engagement scores. What do you think the average measures are? Most companies find that less than half of their staff are engaged.

AON Hewitt define employee engagement as "The level of employee's psychological investment in their organisation". Their 2016 Trends in Global Employee Engagement report was measured with a Say, Stay, Strive model. Employees were asked:

- If they "Say" positive things about their organisation and act as advocates.
- If they intend to "Stay" at their organisation for a long time.
- If they "Strive" to give their best efforts to help the organisation succeed.

This study used data from over three million employee responses in 2014, and more than four million in 2015, across 60 different industries and various sizes of organisations.

They found that employee engagement is on the rise from 62% to 65%, but there is strong country volatility.

This Aon Hewitt study measures six key areas of engagement:

1. Brand (reputation, EVP- employee value proposition and corporate responsibility)
2. Leadership (senior leadership, BU – business as usual leadership)
3. Performance (career opportunities, learning and development, performance management, people management and rewards and recognition)
4. Company Practices (communication, customer focus, diversity and inclusion, enabling infrastructure and talent and staffing)
5. The Basics (benefits, job security, safety, work environment, work/life balance)
6. The Work (collaboration, empowerment /autonomy and work tasks)

While we won't be tackling every one of the above elements in such a specific way, we certainly aim to improve aspects of all of the above throughout our TREAD programme.

More human resources teams are developing their own skills in providing neuroscience-based performance training to their teams through our licenses and train-the-trainer programmes. One team at a large trading organisation is incredibly excited to learn these strategies, and then deliver them to others. I am working with Australia's largest telecommunications company to develop their own internally-led neuroscience of performance programme that has been presented to all of their senior leaders as part of a leadership development programme.

As another example, a clothing and manufacturing organisation we worked with wanted to upskill the HR team to support the business managers with their people challenges. Instead of the traditional approach of solving their challenges for them, the HR professional coached the business managers to solve their own people challenges, giving them ownership of the problem-solving and supporting their insights in this area.

One bank I am working with has recognised that to be ahead of their competition, their finance and wealth advisors need to be more oriented to understanding their client's goals more holistically. They are building better capabilities in partnering their clients in solutions, rather than just providing them with their technical knowledge and strategies.

CHAPTER TWELVE

Emotion contagion

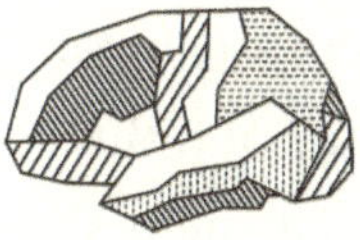

How much do emotions matter in the workplace?

To answer the question, let's see what Tony Schwartz, CEO of The Energy Project, said in an article in the Harvard Business Review. "The emotions people bring to work are as important as their cognitive skills, and especially so for leaders."

Because it's not possible to check our emotions in at the door when we get to work — even when that's expected — it pays to be aware of what we're feeling in any given moment. You can't change what you don't notice. Negative emotions spread fast and they're highly toxic.'[33] We call this emotion contagion.

In addition, according to a study by Macquarie University, ANU, Australian School of Business of 5400 executives, people in high-performance workplaces experience feeling more valued, proud, optimistic, cheerful, and loved than those in low performing workplaces. People experience feeling more anxious, worried, depressed, inadequate, and fearful in low performing workplaces. There seems to be a very strong link between the emotions that people are feeling and the outcomes of the business.

Management scholars Sigal Barsade and Olivia A. O'Neill, writing in the Harvard Business Review, note:"Emotional culture is shaped by how all employees—from the highest echelons to the front lines—conduct themselves day in and day out. But it's up to senior leaders to establish which emotions will help the organization thrive, model those emotions, and reward others for doing the same. Companies in which they do this have a lot to gain."[34]

Emotional contagion refers to a tendency for two or more individuals to emotionally 'converge'. We are influenced by each other. We have a capacity to automatically mimic and synchronize our expressions, voices and even the way we sit and move with those people around us. Elaine Hatfield, an American social psychologist and founder of the study of relationship science, has done extensive work in this area.

Antonio Damasio, professor of neuroscience at the University of Southern California, says in his book Descartes' Error, "We are not thinking machines. We are feeling machines that think." I would suggest that we add the word "sometimes" to the end of that quote.

Everything in our brains happens emotionally before it happens cognitively. These emotions first come non-consciously.

Dr Evian Gordon, a neuroscientist I've had the opportunity to work with, describes how emotions come first in the brain. At eight milliseconds, the stimulus hits the middle section of the brain — the emotional centre — before it hits the prefrontal cortex. In some organisations, leaders say to their staff: "Let's just leave our emotions at the door" or "Let's just leave emotions out of this conversation."

That is physically impossible. That doesn't mean that we can't put them aside, or recognise them and move on. However, we cannot shut down emotions. They are going to play a role in every decision, every behaviour, and every part of our performance. Emotions are at the heart of being human. It's not just your thinking that drives how you perform, there is a large component of your emotions that drives outcomes.

Emotions are processed quickly and occur non-consciously. Then they feed-forward in to our prefrontal cortex. It is only once they are there that we have enough cognition to give them a name, a label: "I'm feeling angry." We can't name an emotion until we are conscious of it. Only now can we regulate that emotion by feeding our thoughts back to the amygdala – the part of the brain in which our emotions are initially processed.

Even when the amygdala is experiencing a hijack, saying "Aarrrghhh, this is terrible!", the prefrontal cortex has the option of thinking and deciding on a different reaction. I like to think that once we understand the different structures in our brain, we can have a conversation with our amygdala. We can say, "Thank you very much, amygdala, I hear you. Now could you calm down please, so I can get myself out of this pickle." Or our prefrontal cortex is overcome by emotion and we might say: "You are right, amygdala, this is a terrible disaster. My life is over and I will never be able to feed my family again. Time to run or fight!"

That's how, essentially, our brains work: Our amygdala 'screams', and our prefrontal cortex has the option of saying 'Thank you, calm down' or 'Yeah, you're right', and allowing the amygdala to stay aroused and ready to flee, fight or freeze. It's just that we usually let it happen unknowingly, without making a choice between these options.

As we looked at earlier in REGULATE, we make great progress when we can replace anxiety with optimistic imagination questions: "If things could be different, what would you wish this outcome could be?" Optimism can help displace fear from the amygdala.[35]

The problem here is that emotions are contagious at the non-conscious level. A Harvard study showed that they are contagious up to three degrees of separation, non-consciously.[36] I can make you happy or angry, you can make someone else happy or angry, and they can make someone else happy or angry, all without being consciously aware that we have done it.

An article in the Washington Post described some heart-warming research along these lines. A study of more than 4,700 people over 20 years found that people who are happy or become happy boost the chances that someone they know will be happy. The power of happiness can also span another degree of separation, elevating the mood of that person's friends, relatives or those close by.

Unhappiness also seemed to be contagious, but not as strongly. Rob Stein writes about this in Happiness Can Spread Among People Like a Contagion.[37] An unhappy connection increased the chances of being unhappy by about 7 percent on average, while a happy connection increased the chances of being happy by about 9 percent. The study also noted that while having more friends is important for a person's happiness, the benefit of having more friends appears to be cancelled out if they are unhappy.

What does this mean for our leadership? It means that whatever we are feeling may be being transmitted to our team members. If we are in a threat state, we may put others in a threat state without consciously knowing that we are doing so.

That is why it is so important for us to be able to recognise what state we are in and regulate it if necessary. We can also actively help people feel more positive by being positive ourselves.

Goleman, in his article on the biology of leadership in the Harvard Business Review, outlines some important implications of having higher social intelligence. The outcomes can be as diverse as less emotional exhaustion and a 6% increase in sales.[38] Furthermore, he also describes how top performing leaders elicited laughter from their subordinates three times as often, on average, as did mid-performing leaders, and that new C-level executives who had been hired for their self-discipline, drive, and intellect were sometimes later fired for lacking basic social skills.[39]

CHAPTER THIRTEEN

Social motivators

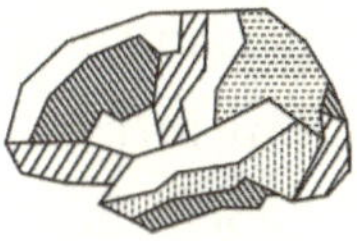

In the last few years, a new understanding of human interaction has come from the field of 'social cognitive neuroscience'. This field addresses the strong relational aspects people have to each other via both conscious and non-conscious pathways in the brain. A leader's ability to motivate, inspire, lead, and manage change with their team is largely dependent on their ability to understand themselves and others in this interaction of social needs.

Dr David Rock, founder of the Neuroleadership Institute, developed a model to help explain these social motivators. This is a well-known model and has been useful to help the leaders I coach understand the dynamics of their interactions with others.

Below I have outlined some social motivators that we learnt about in the Middlesex University Post Graduate studies, as well as input from some neuroscientists I have worked or studied with. If we can access these social motivators we are in a better position to understand the things that will throw the people around us into threat or reward.

As I describe these principles, think about the relevance to you and your work. Abraham Maslow, for example, in his Theory of Human Motivation (published in 1943), presented what has long been accepted as the hierarchical triangle of human needs and motivation. He lists from bottom to top Physiological, Safety, Social, Esteem, and at the summit Self-actualization.[40] In his earlier work, Social was not one of the primary human needs, but rather listed as a secondary need. Since then this idea has been questioned through a greater understanding of the social needs of people.

I will now summarise the key elements to access the social motivators of Autonomy, Certainty, Connection, Equality, Status and Safety.

Autonomy

Daniel Pink, in his extremely popular book Drive: The Amazing Truth About What Motivates Us, identified autonomy as one of the three basic human motivators. He even suggests that the term 'management' be tossed on the linguistic ash heap, arguing that the present era in business calls for a 'renaissance of self-direction'. He discusses further the benefits companies have had from introducing a results-only work environment, where employees have complete autonomy about when they arrive and leave work and where they do their work.[41]

We prefer to make choices for ourselves. That is autonomy. A coaching approach to supporting others to have insights about their way forward is fundamental to leadership success today.

Some of us have a strong autonomy pull, and hate being micromanaged. It's a matter of "I have to do it my way." Others don't mind that much. But we all prefer to have a choice whenever it's possible.

We can give people more choice even when we give them instructions. Think about the difference between saying: "Can you see me sometime before 11am today, whenever it suits?" rather than, "I need to see you at 10am today." Give some choice to ensure people stay in a reward state.

Certainty

Our brain likes to know what is coming next. In a way, it is constantly predicting the future in order to determine if the future looks "safe". The more we are uncertain about the future, the greater we experience a sense of threat.

Brains are hard-wired to better conserve energy, which is why we don't need to think about starting the car any more than driving it. But if the car doesn't start, our brains (via the anterior cingulated cortex) immediately flag an error so that all of our attention becomes focused on this error. In the workplace, a leader needs to provide certainty, to ensure that in team members' brains dopamine, the pleasure neurotransmitter, is being released.

Changing the territories and targets of sales executives, in contrast, can create uncertainty and reduce the team members' ability to perform. Clear communication, fairly adjusted budgets and timely changes can give them greater certainty about dealing with the changes. Sometimes small communications like just knowing whether or not we are doing a good job, and what specifically we are doing right or wrong, can generate certainty in the workplace.

With so much change and disruption in organisations over the last decade, a lot of threat exists for employees.

We are all a little different in our need for certainty. Do you need things to line up? Do you need to know who's doing what, when, and how to go through it? How much is certainty important for you? How important is certainty for the individuals you are leading?

Connection

Connection is a primary social driver for us as humans. The brain is particularly good at social affiliation and distinguishing between 'in' or 'out' group members.[42] Relating to team members is a very important aspect of providing motivation to perform. If a team member does not feel related to their manager or team members, they are less likely to be motivated to perform.

Some of us want to be more connected than other people. There's one guy at your work who comes in on Monday morning saying "Hi, how was your weekend? How are the in-laws? Was it a nice BBQ?" This person enjoys high connection.

There is the other one who says: "Hi. You know that report that we were working on last Thursday? Where are we at? I need a copy of it." This is an example of somebody who has lower connection needs.

Low connection doesn't mean not friendly. It just means they don't need that degree of connection and relating to others. It's just a fact that some people really enjoy relating and communicating in a more personal way in many interactions; some do not have that as a priority. Particularly when they are in work mode, these people are not interested in what they sometimes call "idle chit-chat". To what extent do you have a connection as a social motivator? What about the others in your team?

Equality

People respond very powerfully to equality. Unfair or unequal offers can impact productivity significantly.[43] Equality plays a big role in the workplace and can affect morale and motivation. Specifically, in sales teams, the equitable distribution of resources, territories and feedback can really have an impact on how a sales team functions and performs. Leaders of sales teams need to take extra care to ensure there is equitable distribution of resources, both monetary and non-monetary, to ensure the team remains motivated to perform at their peak. Some of us fight hard for equality and fairness. They might say, "That's not fair. What about my team? We need an equal share." Others have a bit more of an "All's fair in love and war" approach to equity and don't expect it, or fight for it as though it should be a given.

Status

Status is the position an individual occupies, or feels they occupy, relative to another. In nature, the higher the status, the greater the likelihood of longevity.[44] Status nowadays is about showing our achievement. I'm earning more; I got a promotion, and a better one this year than last year; I'm driving a better car, have a bigger home, wear better clothes; all of those are marks of our status. We also measure status against ourselves. For example: "I'm swimming my laps in the pool this week in 43 seconds, whereas last week it took me 46 seconds."

A threat to our status may occur if a colleague is promoted ahead of us in a competitive situation and we perceive our status to be lowered. If the sense of threat persists, particularly if combined with other threats, we become more sensitive to other threats and stresses, and thus become reactive, rather than proactive, to opportunities. The limbic system, protecting our survival, goes on heightened alert for further threats.

For some, status is their driving motivation. These people can be insensitive – particularly when fairness and connectedness are not strong – to others' social pain. People who have a strong status need to focus on self-promotion, development, and advancement. On the other hand, status is a very positive driver for performance, pushing people to succeed and achieve. When a leader is aware of a person's need for status, they can ensure they provide recognition for performance, award structures, and promotional opportunities to keep them engaged and in a reward-focused, 'toward' state.

One aspect of status is that it requires feedback. People who have high status requirements like to be told, "Well done, that was a great report you did." People who are not motivated by increasing their status don't need that feedback as much; they know whether it's good or not. There are also people who are motivated by status, but it's against their own internal measures: "Hey, I've done better, and good on me." A lot of sportspeople are like this; they compare against their personal best. And for some of us, we don't ever measure ourselves against others, or against ourselves, and status is not a driver. So how much is status important to you?

Safety

Safety is about the extent to which we need to feel safe with others. Some of us feel naturally safe with a group of new people, and are quite happy to share the most intimate secrets the first second we meet others. We will more naturally open up. For others, we see people we don't know well as strangers, and only once we get to know them do we feel safe and share a bit more. The safer we feel, the more we share. If you generally feel safe with other people, then it's not something that will throw you into mega threat or reward. But if you have extremely high safety requirements, being put on the spot in front of a group can push you straight into threat state.

Social cognitive motivators

To start to understand these cognitive social motivators, it's important to understand which of these are more important to you personally. What motivates you? A simple way to do this is to rank them from one to six. Which order would you put them in?

We go into a threat state more easily when we encounter our top two or three. Why? Because they are our drivers. However, these may be a different set to our team members and we don't naturally cater for the ones that aren't as important to us. We don't think about them as much as the others. This means we can easily put others into a threat state, unless we are aware of these social cognitive motivators and the relative importance others place on them.

To practice understanding this, share this exercise first with some peers, or your friends and family. Then compare your responses to the responses of others. You can then share this with your team members to gain a better understanding of their drivers. What do you discover from understanding the social motivators that are important for you as a leader? Make some notes to yourself about how well you cater to the social cognitive motivators that aren't as important to you.

PART FOUR
Adapt

CHAPTER FOURTEEN

Neuroplasticity

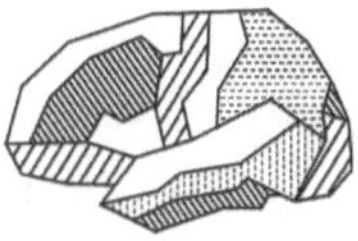

We think that we can't teach an old dog new tricks – that is how the old saying goes. Well, we can! All of us have a brain that is highly plastic. Neuroplasticity – which is the term that describes our brain's ability to change – is the greatest finding in neuroscience in the last 400 years. In fact, neuroscientists say that in the last ten years, we have found out more about the brain than we found in the 400 years prior to that. A big part of that discovery is neuroplasticity.

What does this ability for our brain to change mean for leaders? It means two things: Adapting to change, and changing to adapt. Let me explain those ideas.

Neuroplasticity describes the brain's ability to change; it changes with every single thought we have. The 19th century American physician and poet Oliver Wendell Holmes Jnr once said, "A mind, once stretched by a new idea, never regains its original dimensions." How prescient he was! We are now finding through neuroscience that every single thought we have leaves some material trace. Norman Doidge wrote about this in his book,

The Brain That Changes Itself.[45] It's quite amazing to think that a thought leaves a material trace and changes your brain.

Self-directed neuroplasticity: Can't teach an old dog new tricks?

If neuroplasticity is the brain's ability to change, self-directed neuroplasticity is your ability to change your own brain. If there was one aspect you could change about how your brain works, what would you change? Would it be something that you either procrastinate over or beat yourself up about? Or you are too quick to react to a negative situation? Do you have questions of self-doubt? Everyone has one or two things that they would like to change (if not more!). It could be you are a neat-freak, or it could be you are a messy-freak. Perhaps you have to do things in a particular order, or go a certain way to work every day. The important point is that anything you want to change, you can change. Let me say that again. If you really want to, you can change. So, what does this change involve?

Hebb's Law

Hebb's Law is summarised as "Cells that fire together, wire together". It tells us three important pieces of information about the brain:

1. Existing wiring does not deconstruct
2. We need to create new wiring to achieve change
3. Attention and positive feedback create new wiring

Neurons have long stem-like axons extending out like a starfish or a sea anemone. They meet at the synapse - the space between - the plug-like shape on the end of the axon. This is where the neurochemicals jump from one neuron to the other. In our brain, there are a hundred billion neurons, and each of them has up to a hundred thousand connections.

When we have a nice strong connection, the neurochemicals jump easily from one neuron to another. Let's imagine that these two neurons shown are really strongly connected; this is the "I need chocolate" connection, and it will be triggered every time you are stressed or bored (or whatever emotion is your particular stimulus for the habit of eating chocolate).

If we are interested in changing that habit, we need to create new wiring, a new neural connection that is an alternative to chocolate in the moment we are triggered. Habits, new behaviours, or thoughts can only be realised by creating new wiring, not by deconstructing existing wiring. This is the biggest reason why people fail to break old habits. Don't break an old habit. Make a new one.

From lollies to chamomile tea

I know this all too well from personal experience! I used to have a poor habit of eating lollies when I was tired. My trigger was this: it would be 9 o'clock at night, my brain would be tired, and I'd be thinking "Oh, but I've still got to write this proposal." The automatic follow-on was "Oh, I need a lolly." I'd go to the kitchen, grab two or three lollies, and come back. After a while, anytime

I got stuck in my thinking, the first thing I would think was: "I need a lolly!" It took a while to realise what was happening. Did I really need a lolly? No! I realised that what I really needed was a brain break. But I needed to do something to make that brain break happen. So I switched to "I need chamomile tea." Every time I thought to myself "I need a lolly", I'd get up and make a chamomile tea. I would switch the jug on instead of getting that lolly.

If a manager needs a team member to capture data in a new CRM system, or change a process of product approval, the manager will need to pay regular attention and provide positive feedback to the team member in order to generate this new habit. We often assume that just because we can explain the change, people will do it consistently. We are continuously let down by this, but it's actually a failure to properly reinforce these habits.

The lesson from this is that if we want to make changes, we cannot expect existing wiring to go away. It will not go away. Whatever it is that you have as a habit will stay there. But it will weaken if it gets less and less attention. We need to practice turning our attention to something else. Attention is a positive thing that changes the brain.

CHAPTER FIFTEEN

Mind the GAP

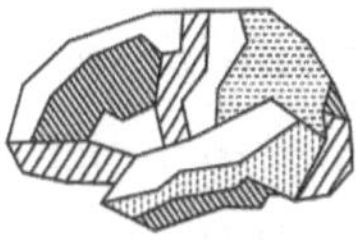

Goal – Attention – Positive Feedback

'Mind the GAP' is the summary model I use to remind us how to change. To become more mindful of what we want to change, and to pay attention to that change, we can start with a goal. Let's use an example of reappraising before responding to a negative situation.

Goal

'I respond in a calm considered way by using 'BLR' (breathe, label, reappraise)'

Attention

Whenever we pay attention, we can change the brain. Each time I find my heart rate rising, I first think BLR to engage in that 30 second exercise, before I respond. One of the ways I supported this to happen through 'attention' was to put a reminder in my phone at 9am every day that said BLR. Even just seeing that phrase in the morning meant it was more readily available as a strategy to me during the day when I did feel the stress response arise.

Positive feedback

Every time I do a good job on whatever my new habit of thinking, behaviour, or emotion is, I also need to give myself positive feedback. If I get frustrated and remember to first breath, label the emotion, and then reappraise (BLR), I also then need to recognise this. I mentally say to myself "Well done, I've managed to calm myself down quickly and get myself out of this challenge."

It sounds a little strange, but it actually helps form the new habit. My brain then craves the positive feedback. You need to know what you're going for, then give attention and positive feedback to it. It is important to measure both where it is now and where you want to be. Celebrate at the small incremental steps instead of only expecting to recognise complete success. In other words, pay attention to the progress, not the final outcome.

Neuroplasticity: The basis of change management

Change is hard. We know this instinctively, and now we understand the science behind it. It's because in order to change something, we have to generate a whole heap of mechanisms within our brain to create new connections. The golden rule for changing any kind of habit or behaviour is to replace it. We have to start small and make it simple. The bigger it is, the harder it is. The longer it takes for us to make the change and the more complex this change is, the more likely it is that we won't do it.

Neuroscientist, Dr Jeffrey Schwartz, wrote a book called You Are Not Your Brain, which helps us understand and engage in self-directed neuroplasticity. If you want to change your own brain to be more successful, more adventurous, and more entrepreneurial, self-directed neuroplasticity is really what you are engaging in. The motivational speakers, mindset shifters, thought leaders, podcasts, and great personal development books out there are helping us to think differently, but we then have to pay attention to that new thinking to make it stick. The whole reason that his book is called You Are Not Your Brain, is because your brain is something you can direct externally. Just because your brain has a low road that says "I need to do this" or "I need to do that", doesn't mean you have to do it. You are not your brain! It just means you've created a short cut or a habit there. Think about all the people who are smokers, and say "I need a cigarette." This goes through their head repeatedly, many times a day. When they try to stop, still all they hear is "I need a cigarette, I need a cigarette, I need a cigarette", so of course they think they need a cigarette. Usually, they go and get one. But if they can convince themselves that they are not their brain, if they can ask themselves if they really want a cigarette for long term health, would they still listen to that message? The answer would most likely be "No, I don't." They have to disassociate the message of "I need a cigarette" with themselves as a person.

The work done by Dr Jeffrey Schwartz shows that even people with strong habits can change them. He has helped hundreds of people with Obsessive Compulsive Disorder. OCD can be a truly debilitating condition. An OCD sufferer might think to themselves: "I need to lock the door", repeatedly. Half an hour later, they're still locking the door. Schwartz helps OCD sufferers to learn that "I need to lock the door" is a deceptive brain message. It's not who you are or what you think you need to do. Schwartz also helped the Hollywood actor, Leonardo DiCaprio, to prepare for his role in Aviator by understanding OCD behaviour.

What we can learn from the fantastic results that Schwartz has achieved is that we all have these habits of thoughts, behaviour, and emotions. We can look out for them, and when we find a habit that we do not want to maintain, we can say "This is not me. I am not my brain. What can I refocus on?"

Helping others to adapt

Now that we know how the brain changes we can get the best out of ourselves and others in organisations. We begin the process of helping whole organisations to change by learning how to change our own habits. The way that we help people to change is to use our knowledge of neuroscience and neuroplasticity to bring about a coaching culture in an organisation. Coaching works so effectively when we are continuously paying attention and providing positive feedback on the progress, thus reinforcing the new habits. We will look at how coaching works in the next part.

CHAPTER SIXTEEN

The mindset to change and learn

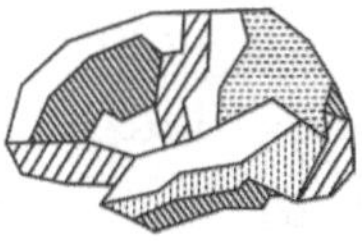

When we change, lead change, improve performance or develop others, we need to start with the right 'mindset'.

In order to change behaviours, or learn new ways of doing things, we first have to be open to the concept of change with a "growth mindset".

Author Carol Dweck in her book, Mindset: How you can Fulfil your Potential, studied the different approaches people, initially children, take to learning. Dweck came up with the idea of two distinct mindsets: a fixed mindset versus a growth mindset.

In Dweck's research, she gave two groups of children problems to solve. When they did the problems, she gave each group different feedback. To the first group of children, she focussed on their ability, with feedback around the children being smart. For example; "Wow, you got [X many] right. That's a really good score. You must be smart at this." To the second group she gave feedback more generally based on effort. "Wow, you got [X many] right. That's a really good score. You must have worked really hard." In other words, some were praised for ability and others for effort.

Then she gave the children another set of problem-solving tasks to do. She told the children that one set was a little bit harder than the last one, and one set was about the same level of difficulty as the previous problems. The children could choose which problems they tried to solve. Which group chose the harder problem set, and which chose the same difficulty level?

The children who were praised for effort and working hard chose the harder set. The children who were praised for being smart wanted to be praised again for being smart. Because they didn't want to risk missing out on that praise, they chose the same level of difficulty. This may seem counter-intuitive to many. When I ask groups this question, we usually see half the people in the room vote that the children praised for their "smarts" chose the harder set of problems.

What can we learn from this? We all want praise and rewards. But the group praised for their effort began to develop a growth mindset – they saw challenges as a way to win praise and reward. The children praised for being smart are displaying fixed mindset. They began to believe that they had a fixed quotient of intelligence. They saw getting the answers right as a way to win praise and reward.

If we praise children for being smart, we can actually hinder them and begin to foster a fixed mindset. We say, "Jimmy, you're so good at maths. Look how smart you are!" So, Jimmy believes he is good at maths; not that he put effort into maths. Therefore, if the maths gets to a harder level and he is not so good at it, he may start to lose interest. This can stop children in their tracks; their performance falls drastically. Carol's research, however, found that training children about how to have a growth mindset improved their performance.

Coaching to develop starts with re-learning how to have a growth mindset. We already know from the science of neuroplasticity that people are capable of a lot more than we first thought. If we give them the opportunity, set goals, pay attention and give them positive feedback, their brain can change. At home, if we change how we speak to the kids and praise the effort they put in, more than their intelligence, it can make a significant difference to their approach to new challenges.

Dweck's research uncovered another fascinating result; 38% of children who were told they were smart, inflated their scores to others. They told others they were smarter than they actually were. This also happened with the children who were praised for effort, but just 13% of these children inflated their score.

Dweck states that "praising children's innate abilities reinforces this mind-set, which can also prevent young athletes or people in the workforce and even marriages from living up to their potential. On the other hand, our studies show that teaching people to have a "growth mind-set," which encourages a focus on "process" (consisting of personal effort and effective strategies) rather than on intelligence or talent, helps make them into high achievers in school and in life".[46]

Mindset at work

The work that we are doing now with some companies is all around creating four key things. It starts with a growth mindset, then minimising threat and maximising reward, generating insights through coaching, and developing new habits through neuroplasticity. Their entire focus in terms of a cultural shift is on those things, which gives an insight into how prominent this idea of mindset has become in the business world.

All of us have a tendency towards either a fixed mindset or a growth mindset. Which do you think you've been showing? It can vary according to our experience. When we tell ourselves, "I can't run"; "I am not creative"; "I'm hopeless at maths", we are reinforcing a fixed mindset. We can also do this with our staff, and with our children, without even realising. It's not great. It is very limiting.

If we have a fixed mindset towards most challenges, we want to look smart so we avoid trying new ideas or approaches. We give up easily, see effort as fruitless, ignore useful feedback, and feel threatened by others' success. That's a fixed mindset.

When we foster a growth mindset, we embrace challenges, persist despite obstacles, see effort as a path to mastery, learn from criticism, and are inspired by others' success.

A growth mindset instead would be "I am continually learning, so if I put some effort into being creative, I will be more creative!" or "I could put some effort into understanding maths and then I'll get more confident at it."

My daughter was saying, "I hate maths and I can't do it" when she was around eight years old. Knowing that a mindset shift was one of the most important things, we engaged in some maths coaching. Within six months, her attitude to her ability, and her confidence, changed.

Personally, I realised that I had a fixed mindset about running. I would say to people "I don't run". At some point, I thought to myself, "Why don't I run? What is this fixed mindset that I have about not running? I have played the centre position in regular netball games. I run. But I think I don't run! I see myself as someone who goes to the gym and never runs. I feel like I can't run."

So, I decided to adopt a growth mindset about running. I embraced the challenge of going in the annual fundraising event, the City to Surf, which is a 14km community fun run, and running the whole thing at two months' notice. I booked it in and said to myself, "Well, let's see if I can run. If I can run the City to Surf with two months' preparation, then I guess I will have to say I can run." And I persisted, despite obstacles. The first thing I had to address was my mindset, then I had to set a goal and bring that to life, and then get into action. It started slowly and I managed only 2km the first few times I attempted running on the treadmill. But after that the more I focussed and shifted my thinking to "I can run if I put in the effort", the more I found it easier to run.

I had one final obstacle: four days before the run, I did the whole 14kms on the treadmill, because I was so nervous I wasn't going to be able to do it in real life. I thought I may as well do it at least once on the treadmill, so that I could be sure I could do it. I pulled some major muscles in my leg, and couldn't walk properly the following two days. I woke up on the morning prepared to have to give it up, but found my leg had significantly improved. I did run on the day, the whole way. I made it to the end and I proved myself wrong. I love running, and I've always run since. I had to challenge myself around my own fixed mindset to get to that point.

I also had a mindset that I couldn't be an entrepreneur. The title scared me. My parents weren't from a business background, so I thought I hadn't even been exposed to that mindset, let alone having it myself. I then thought, "How can I run my own business if I think like that?" Determined to shift my fixed mindset, I bought books on The E-Myth and Awaken the Entrepreneur Within by Michael Gerber. They suggested I find evidence in my past where I had been entrepreneurial. I had convinced my brother to sing at the local shops when we were really young to earn some pocket money from busking. I had started a maths tutoring business when I was fifteen, I ran economic group tutoring when I was seventeen. More recently, I'd bought a house that had a granny flat, well before it was the trendy thing to do, so that I could make some money on the side. Once I had found some small examples of being entrepreneurial, it became easier to shift my thinking to "I can be entrepreneurial!", and that has really supported my ability to run my own business.

I'll admit, I'm still working on the "I don't get computer issues! I'm hopeless at IT." This week I had an IT support specialist come to my office to fix some issues and initially I tuned out, with the fixed mindset of "I don't get it, so it's a waste of time to listen really". When I recognised this, and shifted my perspective, I actually understood much more about what I was learning than I expected.

Identifying fixed mindsets

We all have beliefs that limit us. It's a matter of looking for our fixed mindsets, identifying the beliefs that sit behind them, and challenging them. Here is a list of some that I have encountered during my coaching. You might find some of your own on this list.

"I can't be an entrepreneur, because my parents aren't entrepreneurs. I don't know how to start a business or grow one, I've never grown up with anyone entrepreneurial."

"I'm not good with numbers. I failed maths at school. I prefer someone else to take care of the financial analysis."

"I don't get people. They are too complicated and don't behave how you would expect them to."

"I'm not interested in leadership. I'd prefer to focus on improving my technical skills and leading by example. That will be the main way people learn from me."

"I don't ask personal or 'feeling' questions. That's not me. I don't want to get personal as I don't know how to help people deal with their personal problems."

If we can identify our own limiting beliefs, we can learn how to help our team members' work through theirs. When we hear a person say, "I'm not good at research", we can respond with questions that help to transform that mindset. "If you don't feel you are good at research, what could you do to start getting more comfortable with it? Let's identify the specific issues that get in your way." Or "If you're not confident at formulas or managing spreadsheets, let's pay some attention to that."

This is not about making everybody focus on their weaknesses, nor expecting them to be strong at everything. It's about shifting our mindset and our communication around their capability. We use the growth mindset as the backdrop to our coaching conversation, because we cannot coach anybody effectively with a fixed mindset. We are trying to get the best out of somebody, to help them have insights and to show them how they can be better than they are currently. If they have a fixed mindset, we can't coach them effectively, because neither of us can see the possibility of change.

CHAPTER SEVENTEEN

Adaptive Leadership

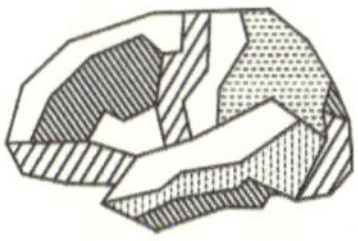

Of great interest in recent years is this concept of Adaptive Leadership. Leaders who are able to be agile and flexible in new environments, that are able to communicate that change, inspire others to come on that journey of change and embed the new changes. They have a growth mindset about their own capabilities as well as those of others.

By understanding how the brain works, we can be far stronger at this concept of Adaptive Leadership. In the last few months alone, I have frequently been asked to speak and facilitate on this topic, as many organisations are experiencing rapid change, continuous uncertainty, and massive threats in their environment.

Adaptive Leadership can be described as, 'How leaders individually and collectively adjust and adapt to the gradual or radical process of change'.

In a recent presentation workshop to 80 senior leaders at a large bank, we focussed on the following Five Traits of Adaptive Leadership

1. Resilience
2. Managing stress levels
3. Mindset reframe
4. Resourceful and Innovative
5. Networking for collaboration

Many of the above aspects we have addressed over various chapters in this book.

The Australian Public Service Commission website has a useful quote on adaptive leadership

> "Ronald Heifetz and his colleagues argue that adaptive leadership is a practice not a theory, defining it as the 'practice of mobilizing people to tackle tough challenges and thrive'. It is a 'distributed leadership' model, which means leadership can be displayed by people across an organisation, not only by those in senior positions or management roles.
>
> ...Management (authority) is best used for technical challenges, problems – routine and complex – where the solution can be found provided you have access to people with the appropriate expertise. Management is about coping with complexity, while leadership is about coping with adaptive challenges that require adaptive change.
>
> ...Adaptive change is uncomfortable; it challenges our most deeply held beliefs and suggests that deeply held values

> are losing relevance, bringing to the surface legitimate but competing perspectives or commitments. This means that adaptive challenges require a different form of leadership behaviour: adaptive leaders do not provide the answers (and do not equate leadership with expertise) and accept that a degree of disequilibrium is needed to sustain adaptive change (rather than minimising conflict and discomfort)."[47]

It is really important to recognise that there is a big difference between technical challenges and adaptive challenges, and that the latter are now far more frequent. Adaptive challenges need an adaptive leadership approach. I think the most crucial point raised is that "Adaptive leaders do not provide the answers (and do not equate leadership with expertise)."

That leads us into the final part of this book: DEVELOP, A brain-based coaching approach to managing change and performance.

As I mentioned at the beginning of this book, the main aim of our organisation is to 'Transform managers into agile leaders of change and performance'. At the heart of this is the ability to coach change and performance, rather than manage it.

PART FIVE
Develop

CHAPTER EIGHTEEN

Developing others – Overview

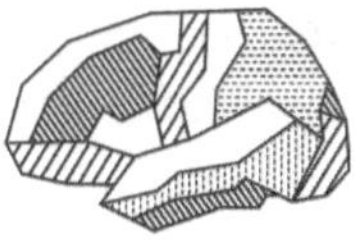

"What we need in leadership is people who are great at facilitating new solutions rather than relying on previous ways. It's quite a different approach for managers who are used to getting better at their area of expertise."[47]

In the previous section on ADAPT we looked at the brain's capacity to change through neuroplasticity. We also saw that, through attention and positive feedback directed towards a goal, we can help ourselves and others change and generate higher performance habits. This next section on DEVELOP is the process of helping people perform at a higher level by identifying what it is they want to capitalise on and what it is they want to develop or change.

Firstly, we need to establish why it's so important that organisations trend towards developing a coaching culture. Then we'll look at the mindset required to successfully develop people, coaching principles, a coaching framework, and finally a coaching rhythm.

In some ways, DEVELOP will draw on each one of the previous parts in order to be able to develop people effectively through coaching.

We will cover DEVELOP in the following sequence:

1. The necessity of a coaching culture
2. Coaching principles
3. Framework for coaching: GROW-WISE
4. Coaching considerations

CHAPTER NINETEEN

The necessity of a coaching culture

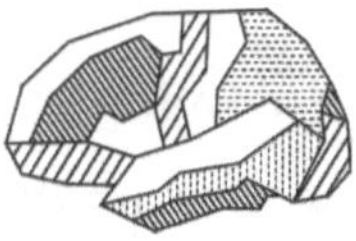

Over the last 10 years of working with companies to develop coaching skills for their managers, there has been a growing awareness of the urgency and scale to which this must occur for any organisation to remain competitive in today's market.

1. Recognition that knowledge workers need autonomy to perform.

2. There is a "War on Talent". Talent is not easy to come by and is easier to lose. Talent wants to know it will be lead, coached, and developed - not managed.

3. Millennials need regular feedback. They are so used to instant feedback from technology that six monthly reviews feel like a lifetime apart.

4. Performance Appraisal programmes reduce productivity and leave development conversations to yearly or half yearly intervals.

5. Change requires attention and positive feedback. Coaching creates the ability for neuroplasticity and change to occur.

6. Innovation is a key criterion to success, and we need ideas to spread bottom up, not top down. The "way we have always done it" is no longer relevant with the speed of change, often even from how it was done just the year prior. Bottom up innovation requires a coaching culture of ask, not tell.

7. Many technical organisations have developed rapidly from a pool of talented technical experts who are now managers. Their natural preference is toward task over people, and tell over ask.

8. Stress and feeling overwhelmed is a huge cost to organisations and to people, and regular check-ins - not only on task management, but also on well-being - are key to sustainability.

9. Up to 75% of people leave their managers, rather than anything about their job or their company. The relationship to the manager is one of the driving factors of performance. A coaching relationship - when done well - adds significant value to the employee. We've all had a great manager and often there was a coaching element to that. We've also all experienced a less than great manager (more usually than the other) and their coaching skills are often what would set these two managers apart.

10. Coaching with compassion actually improves a manager's immune system. When you coach with compassion you

activate the para-sympathetic nervous system and this increases our immunity. This is of course a side benefit, but one that would be welcomed if people were made aware of it.

Coaching Principles

What are some qualities of a great coach? Most of us have been lucky enough to experience great coaching. It might have been from our mum or dad, or a teacher, or our sports coach. It might be a friend, colleague or manager.

Sir John Whitmore was the first person I learnt coaching principles from and below are quotes and key ideas from his book Coaching for Performance.

> "Only when coaching principles govern or underlie all management behaviour and interactions, as they certainly will do in time, will the full force of people's performance potential be released".[48]

Here are some of the other key principles outlined in this book:

1. Coaching is the opposite of directive command and control type management. Great coaching focuses on asking rather than telling.

2. Problems must be resolved at the level beneath the one at which they occur. For example, if somebody doesn't complete an action, we should look at the underlying reasons for this to then resolve the issue.

3. A coach recognises that the internal obstacles are often more daunting than the external ones. Solving obstacles such as fears, limiting beliefs, fixed mindsets, and internal dialogue is the best way to support change.

4. "It may be harder to give up instructing that it is to learn to coach". In my experience this habit of resolving other's problems by providing them solutions is well entrenched and takes extremely mindful leadership to change. Even once managers understand how to coach, are practising using a list of questions, and gain confidence in using those questions, their natural default is still to answer the challenges posed with instruction over enquiry.

5. Coaching can be as effective in a five-minute conversation in the corridor as in a planned hour-long coaching session. One of the key realisations when we train coaching skills to managers is how short a time frame you need to be more of a coach. By simply asking a few effective questions such as "What outcome would you like to achieve?" and "What thinking have you done so far around this?" you support the person's shift into a reward state, and one of empowerment.

6. "We must think of people in terms of their potential, not their past performance". This quote supports the idea of the growth mindset we covered previously. Many managers focus on the results of last week or month as opposed to putting a focus on what a person in their team can potentially create in the following month or year. Focussing on past performance, whether positive or negative, can

reinforce a fixed mindset. For example, a young coaching client I worked with from a major banking corporation was very strong in analysis but hadn't shared that information effectively with his peers. He'd been told "You're good at analysis, but not so good at communicating it with others." We changed that around to "You've put a lot of effort into the analysis and got some good results, right?" He agreed. "What would it look like if you put the same effort in to how to communicate those results to get your objectives met?"

7. "The underlying intent of every coaching interaction is to build the coachee's self-belief". Our job as coaches is to help our coachees see their potential beyond what they are displaying. Often this takes greater self-belief for the coachee. I remember my Thought Leader's mentor challenging my beliefs of where I could get to and by when, and cheekily challenged me to think bigger about my capabilities. I recall thinking, "But how can you say that?" Then I just went for it. I thought, "Well, if he believes that, I guess I can." It was a similar experience with my Economics teacher in Year 11 at Barker College. After failing my first essay assessment in the first week, I asked him for help. Within that same session, he said to me "My prediction is that you will come in the Top 3 for Economics at Barker for the HSC!" While having no real idea how or why he thought it, his belief in me spurred on my own self-belief and I came second in the year. These are coaching moments that live with us forever and shape who we become.

8. "Building awareness and responsibility is the essence of good coaching". Without awareness, people are not able to change or take ownership for their actions and outcomes. Coaching builds awareness by providing effective questions and, importantly, reflective time and space for the coachee to become aware of their thinking, emotions, habits, motives and behaviours. Many of these elements are beneath daily awareness so this can be a powerful change agent in itself. Only once we are aware of our own obstacles in thinking and behaviour do we have the option of choice, reappraisal, influence, change, or control.

I coach a senior manager in a financial institution who, at over 40, has just realised that his strong need for certainty has really limited his opportunities to lead effectively, take on career challenges, and back himself. Once he realised the extent of the impact this has had, he was immediately empowered to address this and create a new language for himself around this fear associated with the 'certainty'. His reappraisal techniques are working very well. His heightened sense of awareness now means that he is no longer unconsciously biased towards creating certainty. Instead he now names it, provides his alternative focus around 'all potential opportunities' and creates new thinking as a result.

A few other coaching principles I focus on:

Coach frequently

Coaching needs to be frequent and regular in order to transform culture. When we have a work-in-progress (WIP) conversation, we can have a coaching session as well. Coach as often as is realistic and workable. For example, every fortnight is what I find works really well. Many of my clients have separate coaching and WIP conversations on either alternating weeks or alternating fortnights.

Coach holistically

By holistic I mean coach the whole person. Not just their activity and list of completed tasks; these are activities that fall into the WIP conversation. In the coaching conversations, we are interested in their motivations, how they feel they are doing, the work they enjoy and don't enjoy, their aspirations, their fears, their drivers. We also coach them around their challenges in thinking or doing. We coach them to think outside the box and have insights around the challenges they face. We hold them to account and question their commitment to activities, we encourage the activities, but more so we encourage the person to be their best. We believe in them more than they can see their own capability. We encourage them to stretch beyond their own thinking. We support them in their obstacles and understand them at a deeper level, rather than just that they have "too much workload".

Coaching holistically means really getting to know the team member – warts and all!

Coach by asking toward the solutions

When someone asks us for help we can either tell them what to do or ask them what they think. We can also either focus our attention towards the problem or we can focus our attention towards the solution. I first came across this concept when I was trained in coaching by Results Coaching Systems in 2003. It has supported my own coaching for many years now. Our tendency as managers is to sit down, ask what the problem is, tell people what the problem really is, and then tell people what the solution is. That is not effective coaching. Coaching is all about asking questions that focus on the solution.

One common trap is we ask too many questions about the problem. Let's say you told me you wanted to be able to "Get more planned and organised, but emails and meetings are running your life." If I responded, "Tell me all about how much you have to do. How many emails do you get? How many meetings and what are they for?", we are focused on the problem.

What if, instead, I asked these questions? "What would great organisation and planning look like for you? What sort of things would you see if you were planned and organised? What will you be able to do that you can't do now?" This makes them think more about increased time on strategy or new projects, less stress, more confidence and greater satisfaction. We are then focusing attention on the ideal outcome, not the problem.

It may be still useful asking one or two questions to clarify the problem, but only enough to understand what the problem is. We then want to focus them towards the solution.

Another common trap is to tell them what the solution is. For example, "You just have to start by putting time in your diary to plan." I start sounding immediately bossy, right? This often generates a threat response. Why? It's not a suitable solution for you. It makes it sound like your lack of planning is the only problem, your lack of discipline, and that will make you defensive. You respond, "I'm not able to put aside regular time to plan, as people just book meetings over the top of it!" We are at a stalemate.

Instead, if we explore it through asking questions, you will not be in a threat state. Maybe I ask you "What could you do to get started?" Then you are free to respond with your own thoughts, such as "I could start by letting my team know not to book over the weekly planning session" or "I probably need to have some discipline around not accepting all meetings, I'm questioning my need to attend them all."

What is the point of this? Quite simply, we don't want to give our solution, but rather ask for theirs.

Watch out for 'quegestions'

A quegestion is a suggestion with a question mark at the end. It is not a question. It's very easy to make this mistake when we first start to coach. When the term and concept was first introduced to me, I realised many of us make too many quegestions. I quickly learned that my "coaching" was full of these quegestions and, actually, that wasn't great coaching!

"Have you thought of ringing around and talking to three other people in your workplace to see if you could implement this?" That's a quegestion. Here's another one: "Why don't you get your manager and we'll sit down and talk about it?" Suggesting what they should do can create a threat state, and it certainly doesn't empower them. We are removing some aspect of autonomy around the solution, and may be suggesting something that is quite different to what the coachee would consider.

The alternative is to keep the questions open-ended and focused on the solution. For example, "What could you do to get people on board with this concept?" Or "What steps do you think you could take, given your need to get more organised?" Most people actually do know some steps they could take to resolve their problems – they're just hard steps or require us to get over our own fears or procrastinations.

Basics of questions

Open questions

What is an open question? An open question asks your coachee to think, and puts them in control of the conversation. It seeks opinions, thoughts and feelings. Open questions start with 'what', 'how', 'why', 'when' and 'where'. We ask open questions all the way through a coaching session, except when we are clarifying, or near the end when we are focussing on getting into action. Often the best questions start with "what" and "how" as they generate the most open form of question.

Closed questions

A closed question usually starts with 'do', 'are', 'does', 'is', 'would', 'could'. These are useful mainly for clarifying. "Do I understand you correctly when you say….?" This is where we tend to be making quegestions a lot. "Could you....", "Do you think you should....?"

Near the end, we can usefully ask "Are you committed to taking some action?'

Questions to avoid

Even though "Why?" is an open question, be mindful that it can create a threat state. We grew up with our parents saying "Why did you hit Johnny?" "Why did you climb the tree, I told you that you might fall down?" When we came home from school, our parents certainly didn't ask, "Why did you get an A in maths?"

So "why" is often not associated with anything positive. If we need to know why, we might ask, "What led you to make that decision?" or "What was your thinking around that?" It still sounds less offensive than "Why would you think that?", "Why wouldn't you do that?" You might ask a direct 'why' question occasionally, but be aware that 'why' can create a threat state.

CHAPTER TWENTY

GROW-WISE: a brain based coaching method

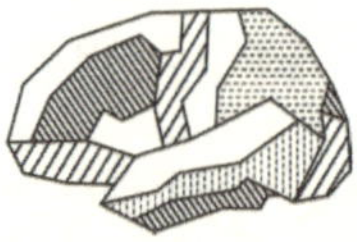

The GROW model is a well-known coaching model, and you may already be familiar with it.

The model was originally developed in the 1980s by performance coach Sir John Whitmore, although other coaches such as Alan Fine and Alexander Graham have also helped to develop it. It was popularized in Sir John's best-selling book, Coaching for Performance. The GROW model of coaching helps us move forward in a conversation. GROW stands for Goal, Reality, Options, What next? It lies at the heart of all the coaching I do and many organisations have trained their managers in GROW to improve coaching conversations.

We can do better. The GROW model is wonderful, but it doesn't go all the way. To fill this gap, we've developed the WISE tail to the model. So let's work through an example of how we use the basic model, followed by how we use the full GROW-WISE model. To make it easy, I am going to use a productivity example.

Using just the GROW model, our conversation would look like this:

GOAL

Q: What do you want to achieve?

A: I want to be more able to influence stakeholders.

It's important to make sure the goal is specific, measureable, achievable, realistic, and time framed (also called a SMART goal). Then we move to R for reality.

REALITY

Qs: Where are you at now? When do you need to influence these stakeholders? How do you do that now? (Only ask one at a time).

A: I currently keep my opinions to myself in certain meetings as I don't think they are interested in my perspective. I mainly try to influence via email and bringing the key facts to the person I'm trying to influence.

It's important to question this person's current reality. Ask enough questions to gain an understanding. What's involved in improving their influencing capability?

OPTIONS:

Qs: What options do you have to continue to influence outside of an email and facts?

A: I could arrange some one-on-one time. I could spend time preparing before the meeting. I could identify who I need to influence more and get to know them better.

WILL/WHAT

Q: Given our conversation, what could you do differently in the next week or two, to ensure you'll move forward?

A: I will make a list of the key people and arrange a one-on-one with them in the next two weeks. I will also do some better preparation prior to our group meetings so that I know I have the correct information with me to raise my concerns.

GROW-WISE

Now I'd like to show you a brain-based approach to the same conversation. In this model, the GROW is more likely above the surface of our consciousness, and the WISE is beneath the surface. As John Whitmore stated:

1. Problems must be resolved at the level beneath the one at which they occur.
2. A coach recognises that the internal obstacles are often more daunting than the external ones.

Imagine we are an iceberg. The part of the iceberg that is above the surface of the water is our conscious awareness. That is all

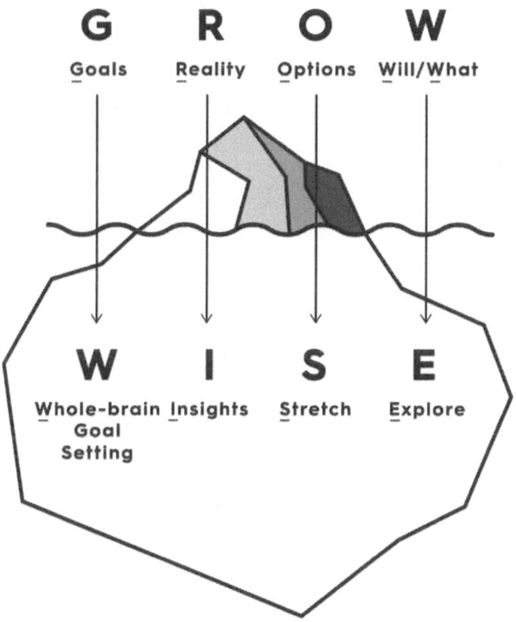

about results, behaviours, and skills. Everything we just described in the GROW model is above the line.

What's beneath the surface is not easily apparent. Motivations, challenges, thinking or feelings around this goal. Beneath the surface is:

Whole-brain goal setting - addressing thinking, imagination, and feeling

Insights - non-conscious connections that we become aware of consciously

Stretch - for the subconscious to be creative and innovative in problem solving and alternatives

Explore - using implementation intentions to get people into committed action

I will briefly explain each of these below, then take deeper look at them with our sample exercise.

Whole-brain goal setting

In business, we have typically set goals using aspects associated with the more left (logical, concrete, sequential, measurable) brain functions. In reality, this means we often don't get the whole brain involved. That includes emotions, visuals, and expressions. Whole-brain goal setting aims to address this and make the goal setting process richer and more involved for the brain, increasing the likelihood of attachment, motivation and achievement.

Engaging our emotions and creative visualisation in goal setting

There is a bit of a lopsided approach with the typical SMART (specific, measurable, attainable, realistic and timely) goals. They are, quite frankly, boring for our brain. When we ask the questions about what they want to achieve, by when, and how will they measure it, your coachee will probably parrot back their answers, with barely a smile. They won't connect: they are just functional statements.

"I'd like to increase my sales by 20% by the end of the year"

While it is important to have these measures and timeframes, it is also important that we engage the brain on a different level. We need to ask questions to arouse the rest of the brain, engaging our emotional and visual centres. These are summarised as SAFE goal setting questions:

See it:	What will it look like? What will you see when you achieve this?
Accept it	Can you imagine achieving that?
Feel it	How will you feel when you achieve it?
Express it	Who will you share this goal with, who will you tell?

Whole brain goal setting is, as the name implies, about using the whole of our brain to set and achieve our goal. We get people inspired by getting them talking about what it will mean to them; that vision serves as the motivator. In this case, the motivators are a healthy mind and body, and a sense of achievement.

Creative visualisation also increases the alpha brainwaves which in turn are more likely to support insight generation.

Insights

If we focus only on the Reality of the current physical situation, we are missing the opportunity to gain Insight around the current thinking about the situation. For example, "Where are you at now?" results in "I'm keep my opinions largely to myself or in writing". This is relevant for the first part of the current situation, but what more would we learn if we were to ask "What thinking are you doing around this?" or "What is going on for you?" We may hear answers like:

> "I don't like to get criticised in public" or
>
> "I find a couple of people intimidating and highly critical"

Both these later answers address the real issue underneath the factual and physical aspects. They are the internal barriers than need to be addressed if any insights will be realised and progress is going to be made.

In order to achieve insights, as we covered in part one of THINK, we need to be in a reflective state to have an insight. Asking people about their thinking makes them reflective. They are looking inwards. Examples of questions here that get people to reflect include "What thinking are you doing about this?", "What thinking do you need to do around this situation?"

If you can translate this into every business problem, so that people aren't just asked what they are going to do but also what are they thinking, they are much more likely to have their own insights. These insights might be about what is really going on for them, what might be stopping them moving forward, as well as innovative ways to reach their goals.

Stretch

When we first ask our coachee about what options they could consider, they usually provide a couple of options retrieved from their prefrontal cortex. We can stretch them by asking "What else?" or "What would someone else consider in this position?" or "What other creative options might there be?" These are not usually easy to answer. They may physically look up and away, non-consciously trying to quieten their brain in order to have an insight to answer this.

This is where our coachees have the opportunity to 'think outside the square' and approach the situation differently to how they would usually. They are often quite motivated from this new idea or a version of it. One great question that really gets people thinking innovatively is "What would Richard Branson do?" People respond with a range of 'big' ideas that aren't entirely feasible. However, the next question is simply: "What is a version of that that you could do? "They can then find new ideas that they may not have otherwise thought of, but that are feasible to their circumstances.

Explore

As a coach, I have found we need to help people become aware of what could get in their way as they move towards their goals. This is about imagining the future, and overcoming barriers. I am not talking about focusing on the negatives, but about being realistic. Many people say they are going to get into action, yet they don't. Why not? Why can't they overcome quite small challenges? I think it's because we don't discuss what thoughts, beliefs, and behaviours might stop them from getting into action.

Their busy life gets in their way, and they haven't prepared to deal with it.

It's worth discussing, "What do you need to overcome for you to move forward here?" If they say, "Nothing stops me!" that is great; go for it. But when we ask this question, we often get answers like, "I end up thinking I'm too busy to have these meetings and I'm unlikely to change their mind anyway." If we don't talk about how our coachees can overcome obstacles, we come back in two weeks and say "How did you go", and they say "Well, I've been too busy to have those meetings… "

There are two key things we address here in Explore. Firstly, set out the detail of what they are going to do and exactly when. It's not usually enough for someone to say they are going to make a few appointments or start prospecting – neither is likely to happen if we don't explore when that would realistically fit in their diary or schedule.

Secondly, as mentioned, a plan to meet with others or do some prospecting is likely to encounter a barrier between the idea and the implementation. The use of implementation intentions is a way of increasing the likelihood of completion.

Research on this by Frank Wieber and Peter Gollwitzer is summarised in their article Overcoming Procrastination through Planning.[49] They say we can use "implementation intentions as an easily applicable planning strategy that can help overcome procrastination by automating action control."

As Wieber and Gollwitzer write, "the control over the initiation of the . . . behaviour is delegated to the specified situation . . . without requiring a second conscious decision." They note in a few places that the most effective form for an implementation intention is the "if . . . then" format.

We start by asking our coachee "What might get in your way of completing this action?" They may say "I'm too busy!" or "My emails pile up and I can't seem to make time to prospect". We then ask using an "If... then" question. "If you think you are going to be too busy to prioritise this, then what can you do?" Our coachee may reply "I could set up the times with these people now, straight after this meeting, then I won't have to make another time to plan them."

Or similarly, if we ask "What will you do to prospect, if your emails are piling up?" They may respond, "I'll start work that day half an hour earlier, only attend to the five most urgent emails, and attend to the others after my prospecting client's session."

We are giving them the tools to problem solve when they hit the inevitable road blocks. We're also giving them the mindset to believe that they can beat these barriers. And that is just as important.

"Obstacles don't have to stop you. If you run into a wall, don't turn around and give up. Figure out how to climb it, go through it, or work around it."

Michael Jordan

We'll now look at an example to see how the original conversation can be expanded on with the WISE component.

Whole-brain goal setting

Let's go back to organisation and planning goal and apply the WISE model.

Q: "So what do you want to achieve?"

A: "I'd like to be more organised and planned."

Q: "When would you like to achieve that by?" (SMART)

A: "By the end of this quarter."

Q: "How will you measure that?" (SMART)

A: "I'd like to have at least 5 hours a week focussed on planning and implementing important projects."

Q: "So what is it going to look like when you are able to achieve this?" (SAFE)

A: "I'll be calmer and have more strategic jobs completed."

Q: "What would that mean for you?" (SAFE)

A: "A greater sense of being in control as more satisfaction!"

Q: "How motivated are you to achieve that?" (SAFE)

A: "Very motivated!"

In this example, once a person engages their emotions and visual aspects of goal achievement, they are much more attached and motivated by their goal.

Research has shown that imagining the outcome in the brain lights up the same neural pathways as doing the activity or outcome, which strengthens the neural connections and makes it easier to achieve. By engaging the brain in thinking about the emotional outcome of the goal achievement, the ventral striatum (responsible for processing the reward state) is aroused via dopamine, making us much more motivated to act.

Insights

Q: "Where are you at now?" (Reality)

A: "I am not spending time on really important long term projects as they are not as urgent as some of the smaller projects due this quarter."

Q: "What thinking have you been doing around that?" (Insights)

A: "That if I don't start them in the next two weeks, there is no way we will meet deadlines. Also no one else is aware of their urgency as they are not due for completion until the end of the year."

Q: "What are the implications of you not getting these prioritised?" (Insights)

A: "It is one of my KPI's and a lot is riding on this project, so it will impact me personally. Also, a large part of next year's budget relies on these being complete, so it will affect the whole organisation."

Stretch

Q: "What options do you have then to move forward?" (OPTIONS)

A: "I've been thinking of putting time aside in my diary and I will also need to let my team know. I could also mention it at the next leadership meeting."

Q: "What else could you do?" and/or "What else haven't you thought of yet?" (STRETCH)

A: "I could aim to get a project team around this, including a couple of my peers. I haven't thought about how to motivate people to get on board?"

Q: "How could you inspire people to join you and be motivated?" (STRETCH)

A: "I could create an 'end-state' picture of our capability once this is complete and the implications across the broader business. I could present that at the next team meeting, rather than just my typical project plan."

"Great, sound like we have a few things here to work on!"

Explore

Q: "What are you going to do as next steps then?"

A: "I will request time in the next leadership team meeting for a presentation on this project. I will also share with my immediate team in our meeting and see who is interested in helping to champion it. I will request that diary entries with "Long-term project" not be booked over and ensure I have at least three of these sessions in my diary starting this week."

Q: "Sounds like a plan! When can you arrange all of this?"

A: "This afternoon before I go home - I'll put it in my diary for 5pm after I finish my finance meeting."

Q: "What might get in your way of completing all of this?" (EXPLORE)

A: "The finance meeting could run over and I do need to leave by 5:45pm to get home tonight."

Q: "If that happens, then how else can you get it planned?" (EXPLORE – "if, then")

A: "I will come in early tomorrow and plan this for 30 mins before my days starts."

GROW-WISE Summary

The strength of questioning using GROW is that it is functional, structural, logical, and progressive. We find that for many, however, their coaching can lack emotional and visual connection to the goal, a deeper perspective, creative insights. The coaching often doesn't deal with the internal barriers and external barriers that get in the way of actions. For those natural at coaching, or if you have done plenty of coaching already, you may already be having the deeper, transformational type of questions as part of your conversations. But if not, it's time to add in WISE.

When we add the WISE questions, the goal becomes more exciting for the coachee, which from an emotion contagion perspective, is very powerful for the relationship between coach and coachee. The conversations stretch the coachee to think outside the square and be more reflective. It also ensures the actions are likely to be completed.

CHAPTER TWENTY-ONE

Coaching Considerations

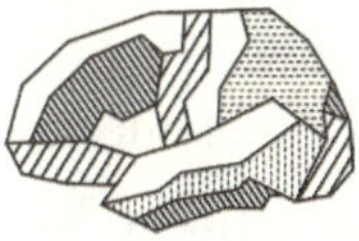

There are a few things we also tend to take into account during training of managers in coaching skills. They include the following:

1. Skill/will equation

2. Peak Performance coaching – coaching for peak performance

3. The social motivators

I will briefly address each of these below.

The Skill/Will Equation

The skill/will equation is a useful recognition that not everybody is in the same coaching situation as each other. Some people have low skill level and low will levels and in some ways, we need to be more directive here. While we can still adopt a coaching approach, we also need to be clear and explicit about our expectations and what needs doing when. When we have a team member who has low skill but high will, (they may be new to the role) we need to guide them more. We need to train and explain! We can't simply rely on asking then what they think they should do. Again, we can still ask what they are learning and how they will apply that and what they can apply from their previous roles that could be relevant.

When we have a team member with high skill but low will (they may have been in the role a long time and potentially could be bored), we need to ask them what might challenge them or are there extra projects or mentoring they might like to take on. Here we have to confront ("What is going on?") and /or inspire ("How can we get use your talents/ skills in a better way?")

Finally, when we have people who are displaying both high skill and high will, this is where we can really take an "ask not tell" approach. We need to remember to continue to develop these people so they stay stimulated and stretched, but are also recognised for their expertise and effort.

I suggest people use the acronym "ANT" to easily remember to Ask Not Tell first" and liken it to the analogy – what better creature than an ANT who manages to get full leverage of their size. If you 'ask not tell' you empower people to perform at much higher levels than if you are continuously directing them.

Peak Performance Coaching

Similarly, operating at peak performance is also a function of challenge and skill level. If the challenge is too high/low and the skill level is too high/low, you need adjustment strategies to get to peak performance.

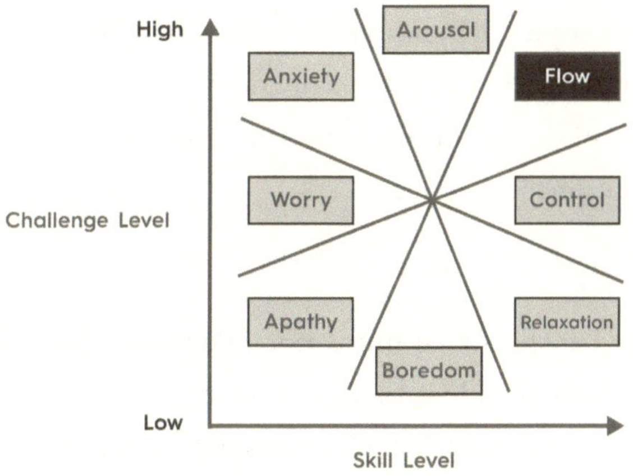

50

The questions you would ask someone for example who is experiencing "anxiety" (could be overall or due to a new technology or legislative change to an aspect of their role) would be different to one experiencing "relaxation".

For someone with low skill, facing high challenge resulting in anxiety, we might be asking more about "How can I support you......... to learn this aspect? Gain more skills? Learn from others? Be mentored? Do some training?" Here the focus is on confidence and skill building. Compare this to someone who has been in the role a long time and has good skills, but finds the challenge of the role/task very low, "How can we use your skills to support others who are challenged? Would you consider mentoring? What else would you like to be doing to contribute?"

We've found that some managers use this diagram to support their coaching to help get people into that "flow" state. This concept is recognising that a different neurochemical mix is being experienced by people depending on their skill level compared to the challenge of the role/task. For some a stretch is more important and for others a calming, supportive approach is necessary, as well as variations in between.

Social motivators

In Chapter 12 we looked at the social motivators. These are the key things that tend to throw people into a threat or reward state through social interaction. They included autonomy, certainty, connectedness, equality, status and safety.

The very nature of coaching is to provide a coachee with all of these. If we ask more than tell, we create autonomy. The person feels more empowered and has a choice about how to improve or complete a task. By them coming up with the best way to address these things they will also experience more certainty. We can support certainty by always being available or adding some additional suggestions where required. A coaching approach genuinely allows us to connect with our team members. They no longer feel like just a cog in the wheel of task completion – they feel valued and connected. As coaching is less directive and more collaborative, it promotes equality. Wherever possible we recommend acknowledgement and the recognition of even small wins, which builds a sense of status. Finally, a greater feeling of safety is generated from regular coaching conversations, where the person knows how they are performing and clear strategies are in place to support their development.

Keeping the social motivators in mind during every coaching conversation, and recognising that people have a different priority when it comes to these (ie some need more autonomy, some more connection, etc), can improve the outcome and the personalised experience of coaching.

Coaching rhythm

In order to really benefit from a coaching approach, it is useful to establish a coaching rhythm. This could consist of a fortnightly meeting of 30-60 minutes with your direct reports. It is important that this is distinct from your "WIP" – or work in progress meeting as the focus of this coaching conversation is centred on their performance, development, career and challenges. Sometimes managers have a half an hour WIP and half an hour coaching (or similar mix) in the same session, sometimes they alternate the focus weekly. Finding a regular rhythm that suits the individual manager and team member will enable the conversation and development areas to continue. New habits can only form, and neural pathways can only strengthen, through attention and positive feedback. This is what will create neuroplasticity.

Success stories of coaching

Over the years I've had the privilege of providing Executive Coaching for hundreds of managers. From CEO's to senior leaders, technical specialists to business owners, and have always found it an inspirational and powerful experience. Through the coaching experience managers have gained promotions, worked in Paris, become healthy, coached their teams to success, dramatically gained in confidence, become more assertive, become more consultative, increased sales, retained talent, increased their productivity, become more resilient, been awarded president of P&C at their children's school, become better parents and partners and much more. Throughout all of these, the common thread has been that people have got to know themselves, stretched their thinking and achieved more of their potential than they previously thought possible. They have fundamentally shifted in their perspective of what is possible to achieve, and become captivated by the power of the mind and brain to overcome challenge or change, become a more empowered version of themselves and much better leaders of others.

Conclusion

The Neuroscience of Leadership as a field has exploded in interest over the last decade. When you support managers at all levels of the organisation in their ability to really understand themselves and the people they work with, the results are outstanding.

As the world speeds up and we have to continuously do more with less, with always-on technology and constant change as the new norms, we need to equip our managers with resilience, coaching and adaptive leadership skills.

NeuroTREAD is a framework summarising the key research on the brain in relation to performance and leadership. It stands for how to Think, Regulate, Engage, Adapt and Develop with the brain in mind.

Research in these areas now helps us make better decisions, understand bias, reduce the tendency to multi-task, have more insights, be more innovative, and be more mindful. We are also better able to regulate emotions, handle stress, and build our resilience. We can engage and motivate our team members in a more individual, as well as collective, way. We can form new high performance habits and help team members do this too, and we can more effectively understand, and lead dynamically through, change. We are able to develop our team members through effective coaching and feedback that places emphasis on empowerment and autonomy, which in turn is more inspiring and innovative.

As we continue to be challenged and challenge our current understanding of how to get the best from ourselves and others, we can ultimately reach the potential we all have to create, support, invent, contribute, lead, motivate, perform and thrive in this ever-changing and challenging world of business and government. I am also humbled by the complexity of the brain and the resource we all have, but are only just starting to understand, in our ability to create better workplaces, relationships and professional and personal experiences.

NeuroTREAD in Leadership Development Programmes

Over the last seven years I've had the opportunity to present the models and ideas from the NeuroTREAD framework to over 7,000 managers in Australia, Asia, New Zealand and the US.

From keynote presentations at leadership conferences, to short one day overviews, from six-month executive coaching series all the way through to nine-month leadership programmes, this neuroscience approach to leadership and performance has had incredibly positive responses.

We have worked with four of the largest banks, large IT, insurance and manufacturing companies, telecommunications, media, law firms, charities, accounting practises, healthcare, education and commercial real estate companies. In government, we have partnered with the Prime Ministers' office, the Department of Defence and various state and local government departments.

We usually work with the most senior leadership teams and their next two to three levels of management. We have also run a number of frontline sales management and emotional intelligence programmes as well.

From our NeuroTREAD programme, a large number of programmes have been developed, inspired both by the challenges in the market as well as the research on the brain.

The following list outlines the programmes we deliver drawn from our TREAD™ framework:

1) **Think:**
   - Strategic Decision-Making
   - Mitigating Unconscious Bias
   - Peak Mental Performance

2) **Regulate:**
   - Stress Management and Resilience

3) **Engage:**
   - Leading with Emotional Intelligence
   - Engaging Leadership
   - Creating High Performance Teamwork

4) **Adapt:**
   - Adaptive Leadership for Challenging Environments

- Agility Leading through Change

5) Develop

- Brain Based Coaching
- Coaching for Managers
- Coaching for High Performance
- Crucial Conversation
- Effective Feedback for Performance

We often team our programmes up with a pre-and post-PRISM Brain Mapping assessment tool. This is the world's first neuroscience based assessment tool and I have conducted and debriefed over 500 senior managers in this in just the last few years. It maps how a leaders' brain is wired and their preferences for innovating, initiating, supporting and coordinating, delivering and focussing, evaluating, and finishing on task. It also measures the leader's mental toughness, emotional intelligence, career development, environmental match and can be tailored to assess leaders utilising their own leadership competencies.

Some of our current and past clients have shared their experience of our programmes below in the following areas:

1. NeuroTREAD programmes
2. Keynote speaking
3. Executive Coaching
4. NeuroTREAD accreditation

Testimonials

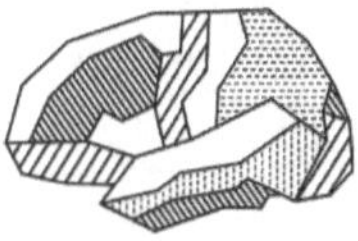

NeuroTREAD Programmes

"I have recently completed a nine-month program of work with Kristen - the program incorporated 1:1 executive coaching, PRISM Brain Mapping and the NeuroTREAD program with our executive team.

The combined approaches provided significant support in my first, long-term executive role in a complex and readily changing organisational environment. I was able to focus on strategies to deal with emerging issues and to continually develop my professional approach to challenges including rapid change, significant staff HR matters, reform and maintaining operational effectiveness. The program also allowed for reflection and insights into my leadership style, my strengths and areas to develop. With this level of support, I was able to manage the complexities of the business and to ensure that I provided appropriate leadership, staff support, mentoring and strategic guidance to the organisation. As a result, my role was insightful, purposeful and had many successful outcomes."

Sarah Caines, A/Regional Director

"Completing the PRISM at the beginning of the 10-month program and then again at the end was ideal, and each Leader was able to see clearly the improvements and knowledge gained and put into practice in that time. Learning the TREAD model, and using the GROW-WISE tool with staff daily and in everyday life, has had a significant impact on our business and we have seen more resilient and confident leaders.

Kristen has made a big contribution to our workplace and has helped shape our Leaders and ready them for future change and improvements in a practical yet effective way, and we have senior Leaders who are working more cohesively and more motivated every day because of it."

Bardha Beluli, Manager, Business Partnerships

"The neuroleadership skills I learned by attending the TREAD workshop have become an essential part of my management style at the Garvan Institute. I gained significant insight into the effect that stress can have on individual performance and productivity, and as a result I feel I am a better leader and manager, and I am more in tune with my team and internal clients. Other significant personal insights I gained include how emotions are contagious and the importance of encouraging the "reward" state in the team. These have all been fabulous skills to learn while operating in a competitive environment which emphasizes excellence in performance as standard."

Christina Hardy

Director – Corporate, Legal and Partnerships

Garvan Institute

"I am pleased to voice my appreciation for the services of Kristen Hansen and her team at EnHansen Performance. As a provider of trade services to the Mining, Transport, Agriculture and Earthmoving Industries we have a team of experienced technicians that have greatly benefited from Kristen's technical approach.

Introducing the concept of Neuroscience of Leadership to a team that can spot the difference between a 5/8 spanner and a 9/16 spanner at 100 yards is not something that is expected to go well! However, with Kristen's clear explanations and interaction, our team of floor up Supervisors and Leading Hands were able to grasp, joke, identify their own and others strengths and weaknesses from a neuroscience point of view.

EnHansen Workshops and Coaching has delivered outstanding results to areas of conflict, identification of triggers and ability to increase teamwork and improve client relations.

From my observations, I found Kristen to excel in supporting people in Goal Setting. She has a great ability to help clearly establish goals and then ensure that are achieved through unwavering focus."

Rusty Russell
Managing Director
Double R Equipment Repairs

Keynote Speaking

Large Australian Bank Group Annual Leadership Conference

"Kristen Hansen presented on the Neuroscience of Leadership to over 150 of our people leaders. Kristen's presentation was engaging, informative and practical.

Kristen was incredibly entertaining and full of energy. She was able to make complex theory simple and easy to understand, whilst also applying it practically for our leaders to take back and use with their teams. The feedback from our people leaders has been exceptional with many stating that they have been able to apply much of what Kristen presented."

Allyson Carlile, Senior Human Resource Director

"The Neuroscience of Leadership training that you provided has enabled me to not only be a better manager to my team, but to relate to, build rapport with and gain trust from clients. This has been extremely useful in my work as a rehabilitation consultant as it has enabled me to get people to trust me and be honest about what they are going through and what their barriers are, which in turn has allowed me to help them more effectively."

Sally Curry, Regional Principal Consultant,
Rehabilitation services

Executive Coaching

"My executive coaching experience was an extremely valuable one. I was surprised at how useful it was for me in terms of developing my own self-awareness, increasing my confidence and being able to develop strategies for my ongoing professional development. My coaching experience has made me aware of how valuable it is to make time for reflection, concentrate on positive aspects of my day, allow myself to feel proud of my achievements and actively seek feedback. These are all things that coaching has helped me develop and have become a normal part of my work."

Alexis Davison

Director Technical and Asset Management Outer Suburban Arterial Roads Program

VicRoads

"A quick note to thank you for identifying and calling the cynical attitude that I brought to our first meeting. As you are aware I was unable to see how six one hour coaching sessions would provide a value for money outcome, especially given that four of those sessions were to be over the phone. I am very appreciative of how you were able to appeal to my engineering background with the analytical and scientific data supporting the neuroscience of leadership. The concepts, theories and leadership models that we discussed have prompted me to be more aware of my (leadership/management) style and how it impacts on others. Overall, I feel that the development I gained from those six one hour sessions has been wonderful".

Julian Govan

Regional Manager - Victoria

SprayLine Road Services

NeuroTREAD Accreditation

"In our organisation, we believe that organisations don't perform, only people do. This highlights the importance of connecting the dots between human interaction and effective leadership practices. Understanding people and the primary organising principle of the brain, equips leaders to lead with influence in order to achieve higher performance organisationally. More importantly, it assists staff to realise their full potential.

The brain based coaching methodology (GROW WISE) allows for improved insights, accountability and motivation. We have found the accreditation process to be valuable in equipping our coaches and leaders with tools that will focus on applying neuroscience to leadership development, change management and brain based coaching."

Anneline Kinnear, Formerly Talent Management Specialist, Human Resources, **QT Mutual Bank**

Postscript

How I became passionate about the neuroscience of leadership

Having been a sales manager for almost 20 years, I was always on the hunt for what would bring about performance improvements in my team. How they could improve their sales process, yes, but more importantly how they managed themselves and their relationship with their clients.

I studied coaching with Dr David Rock's company Results Coaching Systems in 2003 as a way of improving my own sales leadership skills, and found a significant improvement in the performance of my team in the media company I worked for. Many of my team members won annual awards based on sales results, were highly motivated, and regularly promoted. I felt there was a very positive energy among my team members.

I became so fascinated with motivation and performance -- what worked and what didn't – that I decided to leave the full-time corporate life and run my own coaching business. But it wasn't easy. As a significant breadwinner in my family and with two young children, I juggled my roles as mum, part-time sales manager and coach (business, life and executive). When I began attending the Thought Leaders Business School, started by Matt Church and Peter Cook, I realised that to make a success of professional life as a coach, I had to have a niche or specialisation.

Unsure of what to specialise in, I attended dozens of networking events to meet people who could either inspire or hire me. Feeling a little lost one night, I was drawn to a gregarious Dutch lady presenting on 'Tarot reading for Business'. I'll never truly be able to explain that decision. Honestly, I had never placed any value on tarot reading; I prefer evidence-based methods of decision-making. In fact, I thought it was a crazy idea to go to this presentation, but I was drawn to her energy, passion, and promise to help us find answers to our challenging questions about business decisions. And, I admit I have a conscious bias towards Dutch people and their accent - my mum is Dutch, and we have wonderful relatives. Surely this Dutch lady must be good value!

I thought to myself, "Whether this is tarot reading or coaching, I want some of this inspirational lady's input into my next steps!" I arranged a session with her.

I ventured around the back of her property to her little consulting room where I found her in a flowing dress at a small table, inside a room dimly lit by candlelight. Warm and inviting, she soon settled my constant brain narrative of "what on earth am I doing here?" Within minutes I surrendered to the environment and focussed on my job of answering questions and picking cards.

We got to the point regarding the area of specialisation in my business. She asked me some questions about my options and turned a few cards, but what really shifted my thinking were her simple coaching questions. "Out of those options, which gives you the most energy and inspiration?" It was actually an obvious question, but as a great coach, she allowed me to express it out loud myself. "I need to specialise in the neuroscience of leadership and need to start the Masters in Neuroscience of Leadership right away to do that!"

I drove home that evening at 10pm trying not to go above the speed limit in my barely contained excitement. I had made my decision, and although there was a significant cost associated and I wasn't yet making much income from my coaching, I knew my husband would support my decision. It would be the perfect focus for my education and business.

It is ironic, isn't it, that a tarot reading session, a very unscientific means of decision-making, led me on a journey to discover and share the most scientific approach to performance in human history. I won't discount the possible mysteries of life, but in many ways, I put the impact of this event down to the energy, passion and coaching skills of this warm, caring Dutch woman. I started my Masters in the next intake, which began that week through Middlesex University in the United Kingdom, the world's first neuroscience of leadership academic program. I have never looked backed and continue to be spellbound by this incredible field in the science of performance and leadership.

Acknowledgements

There are many people I would like to thank in helping me bring this book to life.

I'd like to thank Dr David Rock as the founder of Results Coaching Systems, the field of Neuroleadership and the Neuroleadership Institute. As one of the lead trainers for some years for the Neuroleadership Institute, I was able to develop both my coaching and facilitation skills as well as deepen my knowledge about the brain.

I'd also like to thank my lecturer in the Post Graduate studies in the Neuroscience of Leadership, Dr Dan Redecki. He made the science understandable and was an engaging lecturer. Other inspiration was Dr Evian Gordon and Dr Jeffrey Schwarz. Both have contributed significantly to the field and to my personal knowledge.

In converting my NeuroTREAD programme into the book TRACTION, I'd also like to thank Diane Harner, a neuroscientist and now accredited TREAD facilitator, who went through my programme to validate the neuroscience that underpins it. To Dian Permana, my virtual assistant, for painstakingly transcribing recordings that helped provide the structure for the book and Ayesha Jahan, who supported me by doing some additional research. Thanks also to my business manager Lisa Baruch, who has made my life easier, and helped with proofreading. It's also been wonderful to work with my sister-in-law, Megan Louis and Danielle Edwards who have been instrumental in bringing together the pieces of the project.

I'd like to thank Kath Walters and Mish Phillips, my editors and book mentors, for their encouragement, excellent coaching and counsel, and for the persistence to finish when I could no longer see the finish line, only a few metres away.

Finally, I'd like to thank my family, without which this book wouldn't have been a reality. My children Amelie and Teo Hansen, now ten and nine, and their father Kay Hansen, have been so supportive and allowed me the time I needed to create the NeuroTREAD programme over the last seven years. A very big thanks also to Paul Blahuta, my great friends, and my parents for supporting me through the last couple of challenging years and giving me the love and impetus to finish my book.

My mother, Yvonne Louis, I'd like to thank for supporting us over the years with the children while I was juggling business opportunities and young kids. My mum is also my inspiration with her own book published called A Brush with Mondrian. My father, Paul Louis, a natural leader, my mum, a passionate teacher and my brother a developer of creative genius, always supported me to follow my passions and to make a difference in the workplace by developing manager's capabilities as leaders.

References

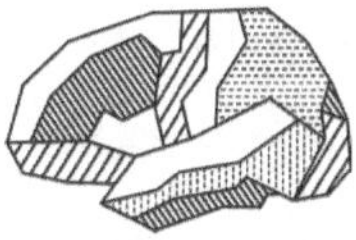

1 http://www.safeworkaustralia.gov.au/sites/swa/media-events/media-releases/pages/mr08042013
2 John Whitmore, Coaching for Performance, 2002, p13.
3 De Valk, Penna Talent Practise, June 2014
4 Source: '*Strategy and Business*'; May 30, 2014; K Favaro, P Karlsson and G Neilson. The Lives and Times of the CEO. https://www.strategy-business.com/feature/00254
5 Arnsten, AF. 2009 Stress signalling pathways that impair prefrontal cortex structure and function. https://www.ncbi.nlm.nih.gov/pubmed/19455173
6 (Wager, Phan, Liberzon, & Taylor, 2003)
7 (Wager, Phan, Liberzon, & Taylor, 2003)
Dr Simon Moss, Approach and Avoidance Motivation
http://www.psych-it.com.au/Psychlopedia/article.asp?id=60
8 www.socolab.de/content/files/Jens%20pubs/friedman_foerster2001.pdf
Implicit Affective Cues and Attentional Tuning: An Integrative Review
Ronald S. Friedman and Jens Förster
Psychol Bull. 2010 Sep; 136(5): 875–893.
9 Brain Sci. 2012 Mar; 2(1): 1–21.
Published online 2011 Dec 27. doi: 10.3390/brainsci2010001
PMCID: PMC4061785
Why the Brain Knows More than We Do: Non-Conscious Representations and Their Role in the Construction of Conscious Experience
Birgitta Dresp-Langley
10 Thinking, Fast and Slow by Daniel Kahneman – review
http://www.theguardian.com/books/2011/dec/13/thinking-fast-slow-daniel-kahneman. **Galen Strawson**
Tuesday 13 December 2011
11 *Thinking Fast, Thinking Slow, Daniel Kahneman*
12 5) Johner Lehrer, How we Decide, p97 2009,
13 This is based on the research done by Amy F.T. Arnsten, Yale Medical School.
14 (2) Kounios, Preparation for insight (brain activity BEFORE each problem predicts insight vs analytic solving). Kounios et al., *Psychological Science*, 2006

15 3) (Jung-Beeman, Neuroleadership Journal)
16 The Aha! Moment: The Neural Basis of Solving Problems with Insight
By John Kounios and Mark Beeman | Nov 11, 2011
17 Neuroscience Provides Fresh Insight Into the 'Aha' Moment (Sunday, February 13, 2011 - by *David Rock)*
18 https://www.transparentcorp.com/products/np/brainwaves.php
19 'Why You Have Your Best Ideas In The Shower', LEO WIDRICH APR 11, 2013
20 Your Creative Brain, Shelley H. Carson.
21 (9) These Are The Long-Term Effects Of Multitasking, Fast Company, cited 8 July 2016
22 Everything You Need To Know About Productivity GREGORY CIOTTI JAN 19, 2013
23 Cal Newport, a professor, scientist, and author of "Deep Work: Rules for Focused Success in a Distracted World."
24 Loehr, J., Schwartz, T. The Power of Full Engagement: Managing Energy, Not Time, Is the Key to High Performance and Personal Renewal
25 Database Reference: Clark RC, Paul RH, Williams LM, Gordon E, et al. (2006); 'Standardized assessment of cognitive functioning during development and aging using an automated touchscreen battery'; *Archives of Clinical Neuropsychology*. Vol 21, p. 449-467.
26 http://theconversation.com/want-to-boost-your-memory-and-mood-take-a-nap-but-keep-it-short-13108
27 Justin Caba; 'Why The 7-Minute Workout Works: High-Intensity Circuit Training'; *Medical Daily,* Apr 29, 2015; http://www.medicaldaily.com/why-7-minute-workout-works-high-intensity-circuit-training-331160
Tara Parker-Pope; 'For a 7-Minute Workout, Try Our New App'; *The New York Times;* October 24, 2014; http://well.blogs.nytimes.com/2014/10/24/for-a-7-minute-workout-download-our-new-app/?_r=0
28 Gretchen Reynolds; 'The Scientific 7-Minute Workout'; *The New York Times Magazine,* May 9, 2013; http://well.blogs.nytimes.com/2013/05/09/the-scientific-7-minute-workout/
Sarah Klein; 'We Tried It: The 7-Minute Workout'; *The Huffington Post*; Aug 12, 2013; http://www.huffingtonpost.com/sarah-klein/we-tried-it-7-minute-workout_b_3416964.html
29 Gomez-Pinilla F, Ying Z, Roy RR, Molteni R, Edgerton VR. Voluntary exercise induces a BDNF-mediated mechanism that promotes neuroplasticity. J Neurophysiol. 2002;88:2187–95. doi: 10.1152/jn.00152.2002. [PubMed] [Cross Ref]
30 Davis CL, Tomporowski PD, McDowell JE, Austin BP, Miller PH, Yanasak NE, et al. Exercise improves executive function and achievement and alters brain activation in overweight children: a randomized, controlled trial. Health Psychol. 2011;30:91. doi: 10.1037/a0021766. [PMC free article] [PubMed] [Cross Ref]
31 Ultradian Rhythms in Prolonged Human Performance
Peretz Lavie, Jacob Zomer, and Daniel Gopher. 1995, Institute of Technology Haifa, Israel
32 https://www.businessinsider.com.au/what-to-know-about-productivity-2013-1?r=US&IR=T
33 Tony Schwartz; 'Emotional Contagion Can Take Down Your Whole Team'; *Har-*

vard Business Review; July 11, 2012; https://hbr.org/2012/07/emotional-contagion-can-ta.html

34 Sigal Barsade and Olivia A. O'Neill; 'Manage Your Emotional Culture'; *Harvard Business Review*; January-February, 2016; https://hbr.org/2016/01/manage-your-emotional-culture&cm_sp=Article-_-Links-_-End%20of%20Page%20Recirculation

35 Srinivasan S. Pillay; 'Chapter 8: Coaching Brain Processes'; *The Neuroscience of Greater Leaders: Your Brain and Business*; P. 237

36 http://news.harvard.edu/gazette/story/2008/12/having-happy-friends-can-make-you-happy/

37 Happiness Can Spread Among People Like a Contagion, Study Indicates
http://www.washingtonpost.com/wp-dyn/content/article/2008/12/04/AR2008120403537.html
By Rob Stein Washington Post, December 5, 2008

38 Daniel Goleman and R. Boyatzis, 'Social Intelligence and the biology of leadership'; *Harvard Business Review*; 2008. 86(9): p.74-81, 136

39 Srinivasan S. Pillay; 'Chapter 3: The Neuroscience of Social Intelligence: Guiding Leaders and Managers to Effective Relationship'; *The Neuroscience of Greater Leaders: Your Brain and Business*; p. 60

40 Deragon. J, *Intrinsic Social Motivation,* The Relationship Economy, October 2010

41 Pink, D. *Drive: The Surprising Truth About What Motivates Us.* Riverhead, December 2009; p. xi,86

42 Mobbs. D, Relatedness, MRC Cognition and Brain Sciences Unit. Neuroscience of Leadership Post Graduate Class, 2010.

43 Srinivasan S. Pillary; Your Brain and Business - The Neuroscience of Great Leaders –; *Chapter 3 The Neuroscience of Social Intelligence*; March 2011, p. 67

44 Marmot, M. *The Status Syndrome: How Social Standing Affects our Health and Longevity,* Times Books, 2004

45 Doidge, Norman; The Brain that Changes Itself. 2007, Viking Press.

46 Dweck, C. 1 Jan 2015, Scientific American "The secret to raising smart kids"
Mindset: How you can Fulfil your Potential.

47 (Australian Public Service Commission, website, last published January 7, 2014)

48 *De Valk, Penna Talent Practise, June 2014*

49 Whitmore, J; p, 5 Coaching for Performance, 1992

50 Frank Wieber and Peter Gollwitzer. 2010. Overcoming Procrastination through Planning, pg 190.
https://nyuscholars.nyu.edu/en/publications/overcoming-procrastination-through-planning

51 Adapted from Csikszentmihalyi, 1990.

Made in United States
Troutdale, OR
11/03/2026

56847402R00132